Bwbeil

D0294152

Understanding

SKIN
& SUNLIGHT

Professor John Hawk and
Dr Jane McGregor

Published by Family Doctor Publications Limited
in association with the British Medical Association

IMPORTANT NOTICE

This book is intended not as a substitute for personal medical advice but as a supplement to that advice for the patient who wishes to understand more about his or her condition.

Before taking any form of treatment YOU SHOULD ALWAYS CONSULT YOUR MEDICAL PRACTITIONER

In particular (without limit) you should note that advances in medical science occur rapidly and some of the information about drugs and treatment contained in this booklet may very soon be out of date.

Family Doctor Publications, 10 Butchers Row, Banbury, Oxon OX16 8JH

Medical Editor: Dr Tony Smith
Consultant Editor: Chris McLaughlin
Cover Artist: Dave Eastbury
Medical Artist: Peter Cox Associates
Design: MPG Design, Blandford Forum, Dorset
Printing: Reflex Litho, Thetford, Norfolk, using acid-free paper

ISBN: 1 898205 48 5

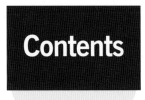

Contents

Introduction

Warnings by doctors that sunlight and sunbathing can be dangerous are comparatively new. Only in the past 20 or so years have health educators tried to discourage people from exposing their bodies to too much sunlight; until then, a suntan was seen by many people as a sign of good health. Even now, some people prefer to ignore warnings about sunbathing because they enjoy it and believe that a tan makes them feel and look better, so they try to make the most of fine days by getting out in the sun as much as possible. However, the truth is that too much exposure to the sun is not good for our skins. In fact, a suntan is actually visible evidence of permanent damage which may ultimately lead to the development of skin ageing and cancer.

The aim of this booklet is to explain how the action of sunlight on your skin leads to these changes, causing both short- and long-term damage, and to give practical advice on how to prevent such injury. Following this advice doesn't mean denying yourself the delights of sunshine altogether, but rather will help you to enjoy them more safely.

Our taste for a suntan is relatively new: as recently as 100 years ago most people wanted a pale skin. Working people who spent their days out of doors became tanned and weather-beaten; the rich and fashionable preferred to avoid sunlight, wearing large hats and carrying sunshades, and saw pale complexions as a social and fashion asset. Northern Europeans certainly visited the south of France and Italy to escape the worst of their winter, but they still avoided the Mediterranean sun during the summer months.

Attitudes began to change in the 1930s as people started to enjoy outdoor recreations more – walking, camping and cycling, for example – and a suntan gradually became desirable for many of both sexes. After World War II, cheap package holidays allowed more and more people to spend a couple of weeks soaking up the sun on Mediterranean shores, and beaches became even more popular holiday destinations in the USA, Australasia and South Africa.

It was around this time in Australia, however, that alarms were eventually sounded, attention being drawn to the high rate of skin cancers in white-skinned people living in Queensland, although European researchers had mentioned the possibility of such problems since the start of the twentieth century. Public health campaigns were started to encourage people to avoid too much exposure to strong sunlight, to use sunscreens, and to learn to recognise skin cancers at an early stage. Evidence from around the world also showed that skin cancers, and melanoma in particular, were rapidly becoming more common, doubling in frequency every 12 years or so; yet many people still chose to ignore these warnings. In

the last two decades, there have also been ever-increasing suggestions that depletion of the ozone layer by atmospheric pollution is leading steadily to sunlight becoming even more dangerous; scientists are not yet certain that this is true but it will become so if we do not take more care from now on.

Repeated exposure to sunlight causes skin photoageing – dryness, brown and red blotchiness, sagging and wrinkling – especially in people with fair complexions. In addition, it may lead to skin cancers, which are now one of the most common cancers worldwide. There are some 40,000 new cases each year in the UK, including about 4,000 cases of malignant melanoma, which is responsible for about 75 per cent of the 2,000 annual deaths from skin cancer. It is also an especially significant cause of death in those aged 26 to 35 who are otherwise relatively healthy, yet doctors estimate that around 90 per cent of all skin cancers are potentially preventable by taking care in the sun.

Later chapters in this book describe how you can recognise skin cancer in its early stages, when treatment is extremely likely to be successful. Advice is also given about the prevention of such cancers, as well as of sunburn and photoageing, and about the value of sunscreens. It is especially important to protect your children against the sun (see page 46), because they are unaware of its dangers, and exposure in early life is thought likely to play a relatively more important part in the later development of skin cancers.

Sunlight does, however, lift the spirits hugely, especially after a long dark winter, but the rays responsible for this are probably not the damaging ultraviolet ones, but rather those usually safe ones that bring warmth and light. The advice in this book is therefore intended to help you to enjoy the great psychological and other benefits of sunshine without suffering its hidden harmful effects.

KEY POINTS

✓ Too much exposure to the sun is not good for your skin

✓ A suntan is visible evidence of permanent skin damage that may lead to the development of skin ageing and cancer

✓ It is especially important to protect children as exposure in early life is thought likely to play a relatively greater part in the later development of skin cancer

✓ Sunlight lifts the spirits and brings great psychological and other benefits, but largely through its warmth and visible appearance and not through sunbathing

Solar radiation

WHAT IS SUNLIGHT?

Sunlight is so-called electro-magnetic radiation energy of many different wavelengths emitted by the sun; it travels through space at the enormous speed of 186,000 miles per second. Such energy provides us with the heat and light we need to live, as well as delivering damaging ultraviolet (UV) rays. The way in which this radiation affects us depends on its wave-length, which determines how it is absorbed by molecules in different tissues. These tissues include those in the eye that are responsible for vision and those in the skin, which are both susceptible to UV injury. In addition, there are a host of other solar rays, such as cosmic rays, gamma rays, X-rays and radio-frequency radiation, but these are present in too small quantities at the surface of the Earth or of too low an energy to affect the health of our skin.

When these rays penetrate the Earth's atmosphere, they are modified in various ways. For example, visible light is scattered by atmospheric oxygen and nitrogen molecules in such a way that it makes the sky look blue; in addition, some of the overall radiation energy is absorbed and some reflected back into space by these molecules as well as by atmospheric water vapour, dust particles and other constituents. The result is that only about two-thirds of the solar energy arriving at the surface of the atmosphere pene-trates to ground level, and is made up of about 5 per cent UV, 40 per cent visible and 55 per cent infrared radiation.

WHY SUNLIGHT IS IMPORTANT

The energy from sunlight has been essential for the evolution of life on Earth. It has provided visible light

SOLAR RAYS

Category	Wavelength (nanometres, nm)	Relevance to life on earth
Cosmic rays	0.000001	Dangerous and potentially cancer-producing, but penetrate to Earth only in insignificant amounts
Gamma rays	0.0001	Dangerous and potentially cancer-producing, but penetrate to Earth only in insignificant amounts
X-rays	0.01	Dangerous and potentially cancer-producing, but penetrate to Earth only in insignificant amounts; also used artificially in medicine
Ultraviolet (UV) radiation	100–400	Causes short- and long-term damage to exposed living matter, particularly, in humans, sunburn, photoageing and cancer of the skin
Visible light	400–800	Allows us to see; enables plants to create food molecules; drives human biorhythms; lifts human mood
Infrared radiation	800–17,000	Warms our bodies
Radiofrequency radiation	100,000,000	Harmless and of no known significant effect; used artificially for tele-communications

for photosynthesis, the process by which plants use such energy to grow and eventually provide food for other creatures via the food chain. In addition, its infrared rays have given us the warmth we need to live, while visible light is the part of the spectrum that our eyes need

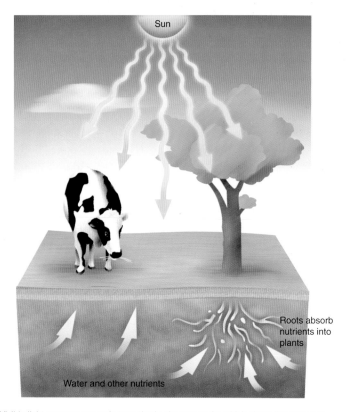

Visible light energy powers photosynthesis, the process by which plants live and grow.

to see, and the part that drives our biological, so-called circadian, rhythms. Our mood and sense of well-being may also be affected by visible light; deprivation of bright light can cause a type of winter depression known as seasonal affective disorder (SAD).

Very small amounts of UV radiation also promote the synthesis of vitamin D in the skin, which strengthens bones and thereby prevents rickets. However, vitamin D also comes in our diet – for example, from fish oils, some meats eggs and dairy products which usually provide all we need. Overall, it therefore seems that the UV radiation part of the spectrum may not be of any value to us at all, but instead is just responsible for most of the harmful effects associated with sun exposure, such as skin sunburn, photoageing and cancer. However, UV radiation is also sometimes used by doctors to treat skin conditions if nothing else is effective, although some damage to the normal skin still occurs during that therapy.

UV RADIATION

The UV radiation component of sunlight is small but biologically important, consisting of the wavelengths between 100 and 400 nanometres (nm). These are then further subdivided into three categories:

- UVC: 100–290 nm
- UVB: 290–320 nm
- UVA: 320–400 nm.

UVC is completely absorbed by ozone in the atmosphere and does not penetrate to ground level, so the solar UV radiation that reaches us consists only of UVB (up to about five per cent) and UVA (95 per cent or more); these percentages are, however, approximate and the relative amounts vary considerably with the time of day and year, latitude and other factors. Although UVB accounts for only a small proportion of the total solar UV radiation, it is nevertheless extremely important because these are the wavelengths that are mainly responsible for causing sunburn, photoageing and cancer of the skin. This is because they are

many times more effective than UVA in causing harmful changes to the genetic material of living cells, namely DNA. As a result, even though UVA comprises about 95 per cent of the total solar UV radiation around midday in summer, it is responsible for only about 10 to 20 per cent of the harmful effects of sun exposure. There is clear evidence, however, that regularly exposing your skin to the high-dose UVA from most sunbeds causes damage similar to that resulting from sunlight, although sunbeds often emit a great deal of UVB as well. UVA also plays an important role in the development of a whole host of abnormal skin rashes caused by the sun (see page 58).

OTHER SOURCES OF UV RADIATION

By far the most important source of UV radiation on Earth is the sun, although the radiation is also emitted artificially by many fluorescent and other lamps, and also by arc welding equipment, and may be an important source of exposure for people who work with them. Special UV radiation lamps are also designed for careful use under medical supervision in skin conditions such as psoriasis and eczema. Many people are further exposed in their workplace or at home to very-low-intensity UV radiation from fluorescent lights. As

HOW UV RADIATION BEHAVES

- UVC (100 to 290 nm) is completely filtered by the ozone layer and does not reach the Earth's surface.

- UVB (290 to 320 nm) makes up about five per cent of the total solar UV radiation around midday in summer, but is responsible for 80 to 90 per cent of sunburn, photoageing and cancer.

- UVA (320 to 400 nm) makes up about 95 per cent of the total solar UV radiation around midday in summer, but accounts for just 10 to 20 per cent of UV-related skin damage; however, it plays an important role in the development of abnormal skin reactions to the sun, the most common of which is polymorphic light eruption, commonly known as prickly heat.

a result of the minimal UV output involved, however, these are not generally believed to cause measurable skin damage. However, tungsten halogen spot lamps are potentially dangerous if used continually, as they can cause sunburn after minutes to an hour or so of exposure and probably have the potential also to cause skin photoageing and perhaps cancer after many years of constant use.

How UV RADIATION LEVELS VARY

The factor that mainly influences the intensity of terrestrial UV radiation is the height of the sun in the sky, which depends on the time of day, season and latitude, whereas altitude, cloud cover, terrain and the amount of sky visible are also modifying factors of less importance.

Time of day

The highest levels of UV radiation in the UK are received in summer within the four hours encompassing the solar zenith (when the sun is at its highest point in the sky), namely between 11:00 and 15:00. At this time, the angle of the sun relative to the Earth's surface is such that sunlight has the shortest distance to travel through the atmosphere and the least opportunity to be absorbed or deflected in transit. As a result, about one-third of the total daily UV radiation is received between 12:00 and 14:00, and three-quarters between 10:00 and 16:00.

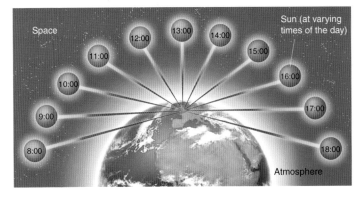

The higher the sun is in the sky, the shorter the distance sunlight has to travel through the atmosphere and the lower the likelihood of the radiation being absorbed or deflected.

The levels of UVB in particular vary significantly during the day, being much more susceptible to the atmosphere's effects than those of UVA and visible light; thus, UVB intensity increases and then decreases by many times between the hours of 10:00 and 16:00 in summer. In practical terms, therefore, this means that the risk of sunburn is greatest around 13:00 in this country, namely when the sun is at its highest, although you still need to keep skin exposure to a minimum between around 11:00 and 15:00 in the summer as radiation levels are persistently high during this period.

CHANGES IN UVA AND UVB LEVELS ON A TYPICAL CLOUDLESS SUMMER DAY*

Time	UVA (%)	UVB (%)	UVC (%)
Sunrise–9:00	60	12.5	0
9:00–11:00	90	20	0
11:00–13:00	95	95	0
13:00	100	100	0
13:00–15:00	95	95	0
15:00–17:00	90	20	0
17:00–sunset	60	12.5	0

*Relative to intensity of UVA and UVB, respectively, at the solar zenith (13:00).

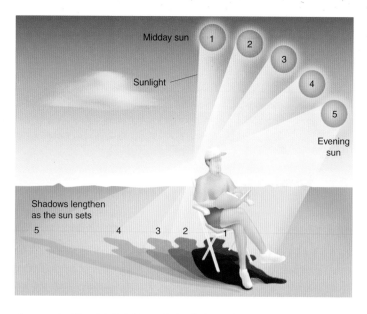

An easy rule of thumb is that, if your shadow is shorter than your height, you shouldn't be exposed to the sun unprotected.

An easy rule of thumb is that, if your shadow is shorter than your height, you shouldn't be exposed to the sun unprotected. Early in the morning and later in the day, however, shadows are longer and there is much less harm from sunlight.

Season

Seasonal variations in UV radiation intensity, particularly of UVB, are most pronounced in temperate climates such as in northern Europe, including the UK. In these regions UVB can vary in strength by up to 25-fold between winter and summer. UVA intensity is, however, more constant, being less susceptible to reflection, scattering and consequent weakening during a longer or shorter passage through the atmosphere.

On the other hand, nearer the equator, UV radiation levels vary much less, being high all year round, because the sun is always relatively high in the sky in the middle of the day, regardless of the time of year.

Geographical latitude

The further you are from the tropics, the less UV radiation there is: the average annual exposure of a person living in Hawaii (20 degrees

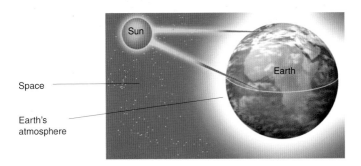

Summer solstice (Northern Hemisphere): UV radiation has the shortest distance to travel through the atmosphere.

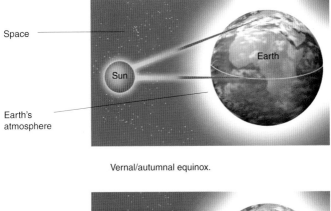

Vernal/autumnal equinox.

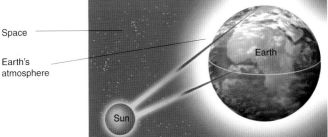

Winter solstice (Northern Hemisphere): UV radiation has the greatest distance to travel through the atmosphere. The further you move from the equator, the greater the seasonal variation in UV radiation intensity. In other words, the shorter the distance that UV radiation has to travel through the atmosphere, the less opportunity it has to be absorbed or scattered in transit.

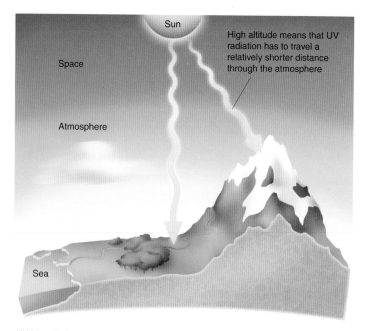

Sun

High altitude means that UV radiation has to travel a relatively shorter distance through the atmosphere

Space

Atmosphere

Sea

UV intensity increases with altitude because of the reduced distance the radiation must travel through the atmosphere.

N) is approximately four times that of someone living in northern Europe (50 degrees N). This again is caused by the increased distance the UV radiation has to travel through the Earth's atmosphere at higher latitudes.

Altitude

As a general rule, for every 300 metres (around 1,000 feet) of increase in altitude, the ability of UV radiation to cause sunburn increases by about four per cent; this is because it passes a shorter distance through the atmosphere to reach high-altitude regions.

Cloud cover

Clouds usually only moderately reduce the amount of UV radiation reaching the ground, having a proportionately much smaller effect than they do on temperature, so you can still burn easily on a cloudy summer's day, even if it feels cool. This is because the water in clouds absorbs heat much better than UV rays.

Thus, scattered clouds in a blue sky make only a small difference to the levels of UVB, although complete light cloud cover can, on occasion, reduce the likelihood of sunburn by about 50 per cent, and very heavy

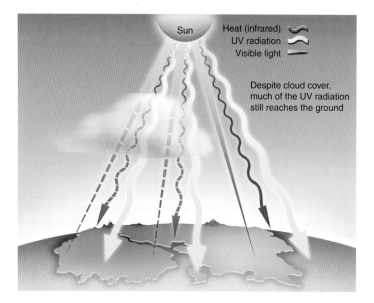

Clouds only moderately reduce the amount of UV radiation reaching the ground – you can still burn on a cloudy summer's day.

cloud by as much as 90 per cent.

In other words, it is still possible to burn in summer even when it is cloudy, cool and dull. Pollution has a similar effect to clouds, again reducing the effects of UV radiation just a little.

Wind

Wind, unless very warm, has the falsely reassuring effect of reducing your skin temperature so that you feel cool even though UVB levels are unchanged. You can therefore get as badly sunburned in a breeze as you can without one. This is even more likely on a cloudy day when you may be unaware of the sun's strength and more likely to stay out longer.

Window glass

Most glass used for windows and car windscreens blocks UVB but not UVA nor, of course, visible light. This means that, although glass markedly reduces the risk of sunburn, it does not prevent UVA-induced skin rashes and long-term damage.

Surface reflection

Some surfaces reflect UV radiation well, allowing more of it to reach your skin and increasing your risk of sunburn. Thus, grass reflects only

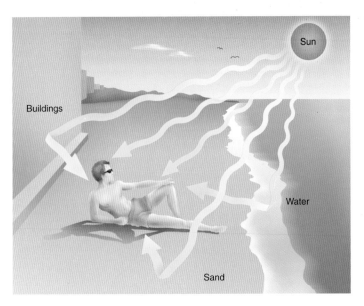

Some surfaces reflect UV radiation well, allowing more of it to reach your skin and increasing your risk of damage.

about three per cent of UVB whereas a dry, white, sandy beach reflects up to about 25 per cent. However, although calm open water reflects no UVB when the sun is high, rippling water and rough seas reflect much more, perhaps up to 20 per cent. This means that you can get sunburned much more quickly on a beach, even under a parasol, or sailing, than in your back garden. This sunburn risk may be increased still further by UV radiation scattering from the sky (see below).

Fresh snow also reflects large amounts of UVB, up to 85 per cent, which, together with the altitude and misleading cooling effects of

wind and weather, accounts for the often severe sunburn experienced by unwary skiers, even in winter.

Temperature
The ambient air temperature (for example, 10°C versus 30°C) or the temperature of any water in which you may be swimming, unless you are on a dive at least several feet below the surface, has little influence on UVB radiation intensity.

Scattering from the sky
UV radiation does not pass smoothly through the Earth's atmosphere, but undergoes many collisions with air molecules on the way, much as snooker balls collide.

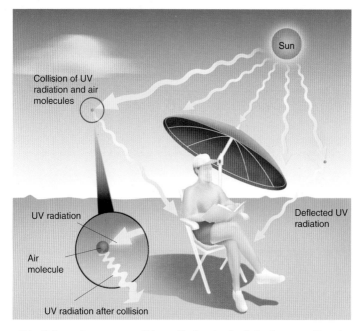

UV radiation undergoes many collisions with air molecules during its passage through the atmosphere. As a result, the rays reach the ground at all angles from the sky.

As a result the rays reach the ground at all angles from the sky. So when you can see lots of sky you are still at risk of burning and other skin damage from UVB, even if well protected from direct sunlight by clouds, trees, buildings or a parasol. Up to two-thirds of the UVB arrives in this way and only about a third to a half in a direct line from the sun. Visible light and heat are much less affected by this process.

OZONE DEPLETION AND SKIN CANCER

Ozone is a gas created from oxygen in the upper atmosphere by solar UVC radiation; the ozone then absorbs more UVC and some UVB, which turns it back to oxygen again. At present, there is a balance between the production and destruction of ozone, the absorption of all UVC and some UVB in the process preventing much noxious radiation from reaching the Earth. If, on the other hand, all this absorbed radiation did reach us, vast numbers of vulnerable single-celled organisms that are part of food chains, such as plankton in the oceans, would very probably die and possibly eventually end all life. While this was threatening,

ENVIRONMENTAL RISK FACTORS FOR SKIN DAMAGE

Several factors influence the intensity of sunlight and its potential to cause skin sunburn, photoageing and cancer:

- Time of day: risk greatest between the hours of 11:00 and 15:00 in the UK, when the sun is highest in the sky

- Time of year: risk greatest during the summer months, when the sun rises higher in the sky

- Geographical latitude: risk greatest near the equator, where the sun always rises high in the sky

- Cloud cover: risk greatest on a cloudless day, although light cloud only mildly reduces this risk; even heavy cloud removes only 50 to 90 per cent of the radiation

- Reflection: risk greatest near UV-reflecting surfaces, including sand, snow and rippling water

- Wind and water: risk not affected by the cooling effect of these

- Amount of sky visible: risk greatest when lots of sky can be seen; up to two-thirds of UVB radiation arrives indirectly at all angles from the atmosphere (scattering) rather than just direct from the sun, so the risk is reduced by only as little as a third if the sun is directly obscured but wide expanses of sky are still visible

however, we would face increased risks of sunburn, photoageing and cancer, although we could significantly reduce these by taking more care outside.

It is now well known that certain chemicals and gases, predominantly synthetic chlorine and fluorine compounds used as aerosol propellants and coolants in fridges, can alter this ozone balance if they escape into the atmosphere and inactivate the ozone. In 1974, when scientists first saw that this was beginning to happen, they also warned about the resultant

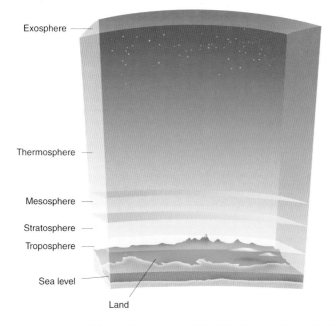

Ozone is a gas that prevents much noxious UV radiation from reaching the Earth's surface. Ozone is produced mainly at tropical and mid-latitudes in the stratosphere.

potential for an increase in UV radiation intensity at the Earth's surface. Now ozone 'holes', areas of relative depletion, have repeatedly been recorded by scientists from the British Antarctic Survey during the South Polar spring; the problem is more severe in this region because of the extreme cold which intensifies the process of inactivation. For the moment, however, ozone loss elsewhere in the world and at other times of year, when UV radiation intensity is high enough to matter, is much less. Nevertheless, there is considerable concern that

the phenomenon may become much more widespread if measures are not rapidly taken to reduce the responsible pollution on a world-wide scale. Fortunately, however, major steps in this direction are indeed now under way.

In summary, despite annual periods of ozone depletion in some parts of the world, particularly the Southern Hemisphere, there has not been a great deal of evidence of any corresponding significant increases in terrestrial UVB levels over the past decades. If the antipollution measures referred to above continue to be adopted, no major increases are now likely; if they are ignored, however, the risk of future problems remains extremely high.

It is therefore clear that other factors have more to do with the rise in the incidence of human skin cancer over the last 50 years than any increased UVB levels as a result of ozone depletion. Of these, probably the most important is that we now spend much more of our increasing leisure time in the sun, although the greater age of our population and improved diagnostic techniques are also likely to be significant.

KEY POINTS

✓ The ozone layer of the atmosphere filters out the solar UV radiation most harmful to living matter

✓ This layer is now being depleted by synthetic chemicals, which can diffuse into the atmosphere

✓ International agreement is currently reducing the use of these chemicals

✓ UV radiation intensity, not yet significantly elevated in populated areas, may be maintained at normal levels by these measures

✓ Other factors are responsible for the present increasing prevalence of sun-induced skin damage, most likely lifestyle changes

How UV radiation affects your skin

YOUR SKIN

The skin is the largest organ of the body, weighing about four kilograms and covering about two square metres. It helps maintain our body temperature, prevents dehydration and protects us relatively effectively from harmful environmental agents, particularly infective organisms (bacteria, viruses, 'germs'), dirt, dust and sunlight. It is also, of course, extremely important in terms of our appearance, and in enabling us to receive sensory input from around us. Finally, it helps to dispose of any organisms that do penetrate and probably also destroys early skin cancers.

Skin is made up of several layers, each having a specific function:

- The stratum corneum: the outermost protective layer, which is a horny strip of inert dead cells created from part of the underlying epidermis; these are continuously rubbed off to be replaced from below.

- The epidermis: a 'brick wall' of cells known as keratinocytes, which gradually move up, mature and die to form the stratum corneum.

- The dermis, which lies beneath the epidermis: a supportive supply layer, carrying sensory nerves and blood vessels to provide the skin with nutrients and oxygen.

- The hypodermis, lying below the dermis: essentially acts as a protective buffer joining the skin to the body itself; it contains connective tissue and fat.

In more detail, the superficial stratum corneum is tough and inert, helps prevent dehydration and protects the underlying living epidermal layers from mild-to-moderate injury, including UV radiation damage and penetration by 'germs'.

The living cells beneath are

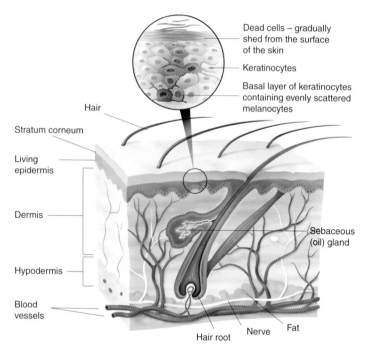

Cross-section of the skin.

of several types, particularly keratinocytes, which form the building blocks of this layer and change as they move upwards to form the stratum corneum. At their base are evenly scattered melanocytes which produce melanin, a UV radiation-absorbing pigment; these give us a tan. A third type of cell is the cells of Langerhans, which are an important part of the skin's defence or immune system against infection and tumours. Like all cells, these keratinocytes, melanocytes and cells of Langerhans have a central nucleus – a headquarters that contains their genetic programming material, or DNA. Damage to this, particularly in those basal cells that continuously divide eventually to form the stratum corneum, is thought to be important in the development of skin ageing and cancer. Such damage is generally caused in the skin by UV radiation, but probably augmented by exposure to various chemicals, particularly cigarette smoke.

The dermis underlies the epidermis and consists of a network of supportive fibres, blood and lymphatic vessels, hair follicles, nerve endings and sweat glands. Collagen and elastin provide the fibrous network that gives strength to this layer, and elasticity, shape and firmness to the skin overall.

Beneath the dermis is the hypodermis, containing loose connective tissue and fat. This essentially binds the skin to the rest of the body, while also providing extra protection against damage from above.

ULTRAVIOLET RADIATION AND THE SKIN

Approximately five per cent of UV radiation hitting the skin is immediately reflected: the remainder passes into the tissue, is scattered and then passes out again, or else is absorbed by molecules in the various layers of the stratum corneum, epidermis and dermis. The short-wavelength UVB (290 to 320 nm) is largely removed in the stratum corneum and living epidermis, particularly by DNA and melanin, whereas the longer UVA (320 to 400 nm) is mostly transmitted to the dermis to be absorbed there, predominantly by the haemoglobin in blood, or else reflected back up and out of the body.

UV radiation has many effects as a result of this absorption by skin molecules, called chromophores; the most important effect is on DNA. After such absorption, this essential structure undergoes a variety of resulting chemical changes, the best recognised resulting in the formation of what are known as pyrimidine dimers. If these are not rapidly repaired, they are highly disruptive to cells, stopping them from functioning normally and hindering cell division. Further, it is now known that even minute amounts of sunlight on the skin, less than required to cause sunburn, can often cause such DNA damage throughout the entire thickness of the epidermis. Fortunately, however, most of this is repaired within hours to days, although a very small legacy of permanent damage generally remains to contribute eventually to skin photoageing and sometimes cancer.

HOW DOES SUNLIGHT CAUSE VISIBLE SKIN DAMAGE?

The absorption of UV radiation by skin chromophores (predominantly of UVB by DNA) and the consequent damage to these are the main cause of later visible skin changes, particularly sunburn, photoageing and cancer. Such damage is in fact initiated at all levels in the skin, but, because UVB is largely absorbed before it reaches the dermis, most of the immediate alterations that we notice are from epidermal injury, although both UVB and UVA do cause deeper

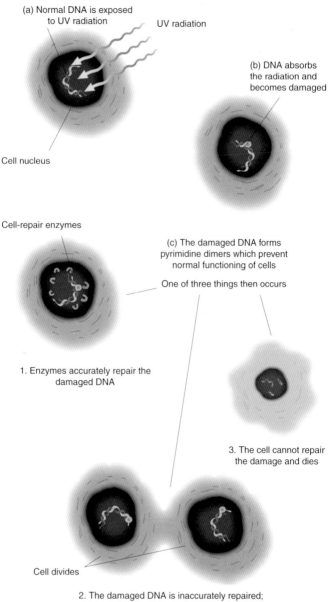

(a) Normal DNA is exposed to UV radiation

UV radiation

Cell nucleus

(b) DNA absorbs the radiation and becomes damaged

Cell-repair enzymes

(c) The damaged DNA forms pyrimidine dimers which prevent normal functioning of cells

One of three things then occurs

1. Enzymes accurately repair the damaged DNA

3. The cell cannot repair the damage and dies

Cell divides

2. The damaged DNA is inaccurately repaired; this mutation is retained when the cell divides

How sunlight causes short- and long-term skin damage.

damage as well.

When skin DNA is damaged by UVB, one of three things happens. The most likely is that the cell accurately repairs the damage by means of a sophisticated and complex series of specialised enzymes. At the same time, chemicals are released that are important in the repair of damage to other skin molecular structures and which as part of that process cause the underlying blood vessels to swell. These events are what we perceive as sunburn, one example of the general tissue repair process of inflammation. The chemicals may also perhaps contribute to damage to collagen and elastin fibres in the dermis, thus helping to accentuate skin ageing, although direct radiation damage to these fibres and nearby DNA probably plays a part as well.

The second possibility, and one that of itself rarely has any serious consequences for the person concerned, is that the damage is so extensive that the cell cannot repair itself and dies. This happens particularly after severe sunburn as, for example, when your skin blisters and peels. However, not all the damaged cells die and those that remain are still likely to leave an important legacy of long-term damage, as below.

Finally, the most serious situation is that the damaged DNA is inaccurately repaired. This results in the insertion of a new and very possibly error-producing piece of DNA into the cell, which is passed on when the cell divides. Such an alteration is called a mutation, and it is the step-wise accumulation of these, mostly in the basal layer of the epidermis, that may eventually lead to skin cancer in susceptible people. In addition, this process, when less important, probably also contributes to skin photoageing.

KEY POINTS

✓ UV radiation readily penetrates skin, especially if fair, and damages molecules, particularly DNA, which are important for correct skin growth and function

✓ This DNA damage is largely repaired, but some persistent abnormalities generally remain

✓ These abnormalities gradually accumulate, leading slowly to skin photoageing or, if vital for controlled growth, skin cancer

Sunburn, tanning and other changes

SUNBURN

The absorption of UV radiation by skin chromophores (see page 21), particularly DNA and the consequent damage, leads to the cascade of events known as sunburn, through which the body largely repairs the defects. It is thought that the DNA damage itself provides the trigger for this process, inducing the release of special chemicals that bring about the typical pain, warmth, redness and swelling, which we all experience some hours after too much sun. The visible aspects are, however, largely the result of blood vessel swelling. In fact, sunburn can vary from a mild tingling and pinkness to severe blistering and loss of skin; in the latter case, you may also feel generally unwell.

UVB is many times more effective than UVA at causing DNA damage, mostly in the epidermis, and is therefore also much more likely to set off the sunburn response. Further, the greater the UV radiation exposure, the worse the sunburn, but just how much damage is done depends on your skin type. Thus, people with darker skins take longer to burn than those who are fair (see below), although everybody is susceptible to some extent.

SKIN TANNING AND THICKENING

Skin tanning

What we see as a suntan is the presence of brown UV radiation-absorbing melanin pigment in the epidermis; this is released into epidermal keratinocytes by the melanocyte cells of the epidermal basal layer within a few hours of damage to their DNA by sunlight. The pigment is partly transferred to the surrounding basal keratinocytes, clumping protectively above their

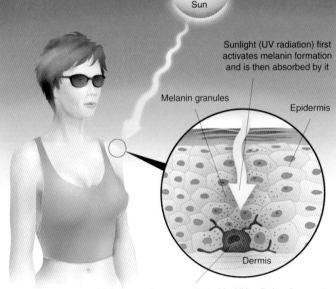

Sun

Sunlight (UV radiation) first activates melanin formation and is then absorbed by it

Melanin granules

Epidermis

Dermis

Melanocytes become activated by UV radiation damage to their DNA and release melanin into surrounding cells

What we see as a suntan is brown UV radiation-absorbing melanin pigment, which is released by melanocytes into the keratinocytes of the epidermis.

important cell nuclei, and partly to the keratinocytes above, which then gradually move to the skin surface in the normal way and are eventually shed. This tanning process provides some two to four times greater protection than before against subsequent UV exposure, until the tan fades as the superficial skin cells are discarded over the ensuing weeks. Nevertheless, the fact is that a sunlight-induced tan is always the result of UV radiation-induced DNA damage and is maintained only as long as such damage continues to occur.

Clearly, therefore, there is no such thing as a completely safe tan other than a fake one or the one that you were born with. Thus, genetically black skin provides around 10 to 15 times better protection against the sun than white, and brown skin about five times better.

Skin thickening

Your skin also becomes thicker within days of sun exposure, and this so-called hyperplasia may last for weeks to months as well. Again this appears to be a response to

DNA injury, this time in basal layer keratinocytes, by UV radiation. Within a day or two, once DNA repair has taken place, these keratinocytes begin to divide and multiply much more rapidly than normal, resulting in a severalfold thickening of the epidermis, particularly of the protective stratum corneum, while the dermis also thickens a little. These extra layers then provide five to ten times better protection against the future effects of the sun, especially for the vulnerable basal epidermal layer. Such thickening is usually more effective than any tan, especially in fair-skinned people. The combination of tanning and thickening together may then give up to around 10 to 40 times more overall protection, much better than a tan alone, albeit always at the expense of some permanent skin damage.

WHO IS AT RISK OF SUNBURN?

Fair-skinned individuals, especially those with freckles and red hair, burn particularly easily in the sun, because of their relative genetic lack of melanin, and sometimes may not tan at all, whereas darker-skinned people do so with relative ease. How well a tan develops is thus

THE SIX SKIN TYPES

Skin type	Characteristics
I	Always burns, rarely tans
II	Usually burns, sometimes tans
III	Sometimes burns, usually tans
IV	Rarely burns, always tans
V	Brown skin, very rarely burns
VI	Black skin, virtually never burns

built into you from birth and depends on which of six arbitrarily defined skin types you have (see box). People with type I, II or III tend to burn easily and tan poorly, being at greatest risk from the adverse long-term effects of sunlight – namely skin photoageing and cancer, whereas those with type IV, V or VI are relatively protected, except for a tendency to photoageing. Your skin type can be readily determined from the way it responds to the first significant exposure to midday summer sun each year.

KEY POINTS

✓ Sunburn is a skin repair process, called inflammation elsewhere in the body, which is initiated by injury; it is produced in the skin by UV damage, very probably to cellular DNA

✓ The redness of sunburn is caused by swelling of the blood vessels used to bring in tissue repair materials; the pain is caused by the swelling and chemicals released

✓ Tanning is the release of UV-protective pigment called melanin into the skin after UV-induced DNA damage; not everyone tans easily

✓ Thickening of the skin also occurs after UV-induced DNA damage; everyone develops skin thickening

✓ Tanning and thickening can give 10 to 40 times the protection against UV damage, but only at the expense of some UV damage to initiate and maintain the process

Photoageing and cancer

PHOTOAGEING

What is it?

There appear to be two major ways in which skin may age. The first is genetically programmed, so-called intrinsic or normal ageing, affecting the skin all over your body. The second is what is known as photoageing and results from the long-term adverse effects of sun exposure. The degree to which skin photoages is also determined genetically to some extent, in that fair-skinned people who burn easily tend to photoage most rapidly. However, it also depends on how much your skin is exposed to sunlight over the years, whether through normal outdoor activities or sunbathing, or both.

It is possible to judge the effects of any photoageing of your skin by comparing the appearance of your hips or buttocks with that of your face. Those areas normally covered by clothing are smooth and freckle- and wrinkle-free. Facial skin, in contrast, may be relatively freckled in susceptible people, namely those with fairer skin, particularly if they have had a lot of previous sun exposure, and, in older people, is often dry, thickened, yellowish, blotched brown, deeply wrinkled and affected by thread veins. Allowing for the normal effects of ageing, the difference between skin that is usually covered and that normally exposed is the result of photoageing of the sun-affected sites.

What causes photoageing?

Photoageing is the result of accumulated skin damage caused by UV radiation over many years. Just as for sunburn, it is the UVB wavelengths that have the greatest effect; however, UVA exposure can also cause changes, although with a tendency to be deeper. These may

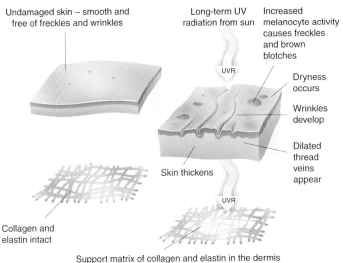

Undamaged skin – smooth and free of freckles and wrinkles

Long-term UV radiation from sun

Increased melanocyte activity causes freckles and brown blotches

UVR

Dryness occurs

Wrinkles develop

Dilated thread veins appear

Skin thickens

Collagen and elastin intact

UVR

Support matrix of collagen and elastin in the dermis is damaged and contributes to wrlnkle formation

Photoageing is the result of accumulated skin damage caused by UV radiation (UVR) over many years.

affect you, particularly if you spend a lot of time on a sunbed or sunbathing using a sunscreen that blocks mostly UVB.

When the body is unable fully to repair damage to the DNA in cells of the epidermis and dermis, their structure deteriorates with changes that seem irreversible. In addition, the chemicals that stimulate the sunburn process appear also to harm the dermis, especially the network of collagen and elastic fibres that forms the major support for the skin and helps to keep it wrinkle-free, although this damage may recover over time; the fibres may also be directly damaged by UV exposure. All this means that

your skin overall tends to become gradually drier, rougher and thicker, and thread veins and wrinkles slowly develop. Sunlight also causes changes to the tanning cells, which gradually stop functioning in a consistent fashion, so your skin may develop a brown blotchiness; it may gradually yellow as well. Finally, your epidermis may become thinner and more fragile. All these changes together are the visible signs of skin photoageing.

Other factors besides sunlight exposure may contribute significantly to skin ageing, including most particularly cigarette smoking, and make the overall skin appearance even worse.

Can photoageing be prevented?

In theory, yes. If you could protect your face from the sun all the time, it should remain relatively young-looking and wrinkle-free into old age. In the past, however, this has usually not happened, particularly because people have not understood the cause of photoageing.

First, it is vital to begin any protection programme very early in life: it has been estimated that up to 50 per cent of our total UV radiation exposure is acquired by the time we reach 18 and 75 per cent by 30; nevertheless, at least we can improve the outlook for our children's skin by acting now. As far as adults are concerned, although the 'time-clock' for photoageing has already been ticking for some time, we can definitely minimise further changes by being careful in the sun from now on.

Second, it seems likely that skin photoageing steadily develops even with recurrent minor UV exposure. Increasing evidence suggests that even walking to and from the office or shops or hanging out the washing may expose our skin to enough sunlight to cause some photoageing. The skin does not need to burn, or even turn pink, for slow permanent damage to take place. This therefore means that preventing photoageing probably requires even more effort with regard to sun protection than sunburn does.

In summary, any steps that you take now to cut down the time you spend outside unprotected will reduce the speed and extent of your eventual skin photoageing, whenever you may start. Although the skin on your face may not look as young as that on your buttocks, it can still look much better than if you did nothing at all to protect it. The younger you are when you start your protection programme, the better your outlook. To do this, you need to reduce the time your skin is exposed even to ordinary daylight each day, rather than simply making sure you don't get sunburned. For this reason, some types of make-up and moisturisers now incorporate sunscreen ingredients and are worthwhile if you normally use such products or are happy to start. For more on the prevention and treatment of sun damage and photoageing, see page 41.

WHAT IS SKIN CANCER?

All cancers appear to be made up of body cells that have gradually deteriorated through sequential damage to their DNA, so as to make them grow independently of the rest of the body and be able to infiltrate other tissues. In doing this, they bypass the usual mechanisms designed to prevent this happening. They are dangerous because not only can they damage and affect the normal structures around them, but also they can often later spread through the bloodstream and lymph vessels to disrupt other parts of the body, continuing to grow in these new sites, which are often vital organs such as the lungs, liver and brain. In the later stages, they also tend to divert the nourishment necessary for the body's normal activity to meet their own requirements.

DNA-damaging agents are known as carcinogens, and include chemicals present, for instance, in tobacco smoke, the constituents of certain foods, the emissions from radioactive substances, certain viruses and, especially, as far as skin cancers are concerned, the UVB and UVA in solar radiation.

There are three main types of skin cancer (or carcinoma) (see box below).

In addition, there are two cancer precursor lesions: the solar (or actinic) keratosis, which may precede squamous cancers, and lentigo maligna, which may predate one form of melanoma, the lentigo maligna melanoma. Basal cell cancers and other melanomas do not have precursors.

Skin cancers are one of the most common cancers worldwide. In the UK alone there are approximately 40,000 new cases each year; of these, about 28,000 are basal cell cancers, 7,000 squamous cell ones and 4,000 to 5,000 malignant melanomas. About 2,000 people die each year from such cancers, around 1,500 of them from melanoma. However, most skin cancers are avoidable and all are generally curable if caught early, which is why dermatologists and health campaigners are currently working hard to increase public awareness of all forms of the condition and its prevention.

Despite these efforts, there has

MAIN TYPES OF SKIN CANCER

- Basal cell cancer or carcinoma (sometimes known as rodent ulcer)

- Squamous cell cancer or carcinoma

together known as non-melanoma skin cancer (or carcinoma)

- Malignant melanoma

still been a very substantial increase in all types of these tumours over the last few decades, with rates doubling approximately every 10 to 12 years. As stated earlier, this may to some extent be the result of improved diagnostic and disease-reporting techniques, but is probably more to do with lifestyle changes in recent years. We now take far more sunshine holidays than we once did, and many people spend much of their leisure time in this country sunbathing. The possible impact of ozone depletion has yet to be felt, but if unchecked this also has the potential to increase skin cancer risk still further, unless the careful measures referred to earlier are reliably implemented. On the other hand, the possible good news is that the annual increases in skin cancer rates appear at last to be slowing, perhaps as a result of the current major efforts at public education.

Basal cell cancers

Basal cell carcinoma is the most common and least aggressive form of skin cancer, developing from the basal layer of the epidermis. This tumour normally grows slowly, often appearing first as a small, flesh-coloured, firm, somewhat pearly nodule, often on the upper face, shoulder or back of an elderly person. It then slowly enlarges until a central area of broken skin

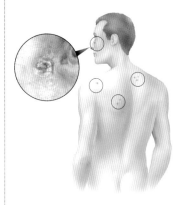

Basal cell cancers.

develops; some people first notice the problem when they scratch the lesion, which may then bleed a little and fail to heal properly. Sunlight clearly plays a part in causing this cancer, but other factors are also important, because not all exposed areas are regularly affected, the backs of the hands particularly being spared. In addition, although people over the age of 50 most commonly develop the disorder, it can also occur in much younger people. The main danger from basal cell cancer is its potential to erode the skin and underlying tissues very gradually but relentlessly over a number of years, although fortunately it almost never spreads to the rest of the body. The treatment is straightforward if undertaken early, however, and is explained on page 51.

Solar (or actinic) keratoses

Solar keratoses result from the early disordered growth of groups of keratinocytes in the epidermis; they generally appear on skin that has been continually exposed to the sun over long periods, such as on the face, ears, backs of hands and scalps of men with thinning hair.

Solar keratoses are very common, as many as a third or more of fair-skinned people over the age of 60 having them, particularly in sunnier climates. They are usually skin patches that are less than a centimetre across, reddish or brownish, scaly or rough, slightly uncomfortable if knocked and sometimes easier to feel than to see. You can check for them by running your fingers or palm of your hand lightly over your exposed skin – they feel slightly rough compared with normal areas. There are of course many other causes for rough skin, but any persistent patches on exposed areas just might be solar keratoses.

Solar keratoses are potential precursors of squamous cell carcinoma, but in practice they only rarely progress in this way; only one to two per cent ever become malignant and some may actually disappear, particularly if sun exposure is minimised. Failing that, however, their treatment is relatively straightforward, by either freezing them or cutting them out, and is detailed on pages 50–1. It is generally worthwhile to have such treatment so as to avoid the slight risk of future squamous cell cancer, as well as to get rid of the often unsightly, slightly sore patches.

Squamous cell cancers

Squamous cell carcinoma is the second most common type of skin cancer; it also develops within the keratinocytes of the epidermis. This disorder is rare in people under 50, and most commonly affects relatively fair-skinned individuals who have been exposed to regular sunlight over long periods of their lives, perhaps because they have lived in very sunny climates, or else worked or had an outdoor hobby for

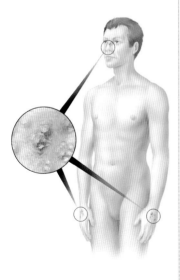

Solar keratoses.

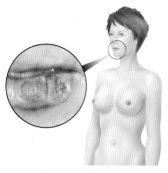

Squamous cell cancer.

many years. Typical lesions are slightly tender, reddish or brownish, slowly growing, persistent lumps on any regularly exposed skin; generally they are more bulky and rougher to the touch than basal cell cancers, unless ulcerated. They generally start off as very small patches, frequently in the form of solar keratoses. You should always consult your doctor about any lump or sore of this type which starts in such a way and fails to heal over weeks to months. The treatment of squamous cell cancers is straight-forward and, except in the latest stages, generally leads to a complete cure (see pages 51–2).

Malignant melanoma

Malignant melanoma is the rarest skin cancer, making up about 10 per cent of the total, but it is also the most dangerous, causing around 75 per cent of all deaths from the cancer. If caught early, however, as with all other skin cancers, it is readily curable, so it is extremely important to look out for and recognise the early signs of this aggressive condition. It consists of a collection of cancerous melano-cytes, the pigment-producing cells of the basal epidermis, and usually appears as a mole larger than about six millimetres across (the size of the blunt end of a pencil), which irregularly enlarges and darkens over several months; consult your doctor promptly if you have any lesion that behaves like this. Many melanomas develop within pre-existing moles, although some also seem to occur in previously normal skin, and the condition is much more likely to affect those who are very fair, tend to freckle easily, already have lots of moles and have been sunburned frequently. Younger age groups mostly get them on the trunk (in men) and lower leg (in women), whereas very elderly people may develop them on the face, in a relatively less aggressive form; this often follows months to years of the presence of an initially harmless, fixed, irregular, brown discoloration called a lentigo, later a lentigo maligna, as mentioned on page 31.

You can develop malignant melanoma at any time, although it is more common in those over 50 and extremely uncommon before the age of 16. In addition, it is still rare overall, affecting only about

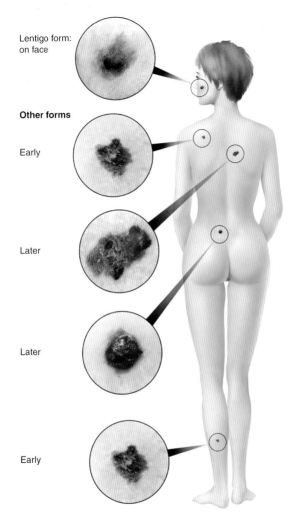

Lentigo form: on face

Other forms

Early

Later

Later

Early

Malignant melanoma.

one in 15,000 people per year in the UK or around 4,000 in total, although rather more of course among those at greater risk.

The so-called ABCDE guide (see page 36) summarises the signs to look out for; these changes often, though not always, occur all together, and continue to progress over weeks to months.

Many people may develop new, harmless, evenly coloured, regularly

ABCDE GUIDE TO MELANOMAS

A = ALTERATION in APPEARANCE of a mole. Ordinary moles do not change, except occasionally for a few days after minor injury. You should therefore consult your doctor if one has permanently altered, particularly if it is continuing to do so; it may have grown darker, bigger or more irregular in outline, or commonly all three.

B = BORDER IRREGULARITY. Ordinary moles generally have well-defined, relatively smooth outlines, whereas melanomas often have irregular or ill-defined edges. Repeated BLEEDING or itching of a mole over more than a week or so, in addition to the other features mentioned above, is a further cause for concern.

C = COLOUR. Ordinary moles are usually evenly pigmented brown with a smooth surface. A suspicious mole, however, has more than one shade of brown, often with an uneven surface texture as well. Thus, it may be light and dark brown in different parts, or rarely even have red, black or white areas instead or as well. The precise colour outlines also tend to change over weeks to months.

D = DIAMETER. Many ordinary moles are smaller than the blunt end of a pencil; however, melanomas are generally at least as large as this, that is, more than about five to six millimetres in diameter.

E = ENLARGEMENT. Ordinary moles do not usually grow in size over weeks to months, whereas melanomas do.

outlined, smallish moles from time to time, particularly around the teenage years, but sometimes much later in life as well. These are generally nothing to worry about, but if you have any doubts at all it is best to consult your doctor, particularly as the treatment for melanoma is very straightforward in the early stages and almost always fully curative; the procedure is explained on pages 52–3.

WHAT CAUSES SKIN CANCER?

There is now little doubt that the most important cause of skin cancer is excessive exposure of the skin to

UV radiation from sunlight, particularly in fair-skinned people.

As with sunburn and photo-ageing, it seems certain that the UVB component of this radiation is the most important contributor. As stated earlier, these rays are well known to damage skin cell DNA, which governs the structure, growth, function and reproduction of cells. If such damage is not repaired accurately, it can sometimes eventually lead to skin cancer, probably through a sequence of changes occurring over a number of years. In addition, UVB exposure may also also reduce the ability of the skin immune system to inhibit the development of early cancers, so that any that are triggered during repeated sun exposure may not be eliminated.

As skin cancer is thought to be a step-wise process, probably requiring at least several separate DNA changes to take place before it develops, there is often a long time lag between any obvious initial damage events, such as getting sunburned in childhood, and the eventual appearance of any cancer. During this period, important additive sun damage probably also takes place. This total time lag may be up to 30 to 50 years, particularly for squamous cell cancers, although it may be less at 10 to 15 years for basal cell cancers and melanomas. The rate of such tumour develop-

ment is clearly also dependent on the amount of continuing sun exposure throughout the days and years, and on the individual's skin type.

Nevertheless, some people who have skin cancer say that they never sunbathe or even go out in the sun at all. This seems to be the case particularly in very fair-skinned individuals and is probably because they are very sun sensitive, and repeated minor exposures in their early lives and young adulthood may have been the major factors in their cancer development. Other people who work or spend a great deal of leisure time outside may simply pay no attention to whether they are in the sun or not. Thus, just as for skin photoageing, the 'time-clock' for skin cancer may be ticking from very early life. Someone who has skin cancer today, for example, may have had a lot of sun while on National Service when young in the Far East, or during a childhood spent on a farm, or perhaps through sunbathing every summer as a teenager or young adult. This is clearly not to say that older people need not worry about sun protection – continuing exposure also appears very important in causing the damage that eventually leads to skin cancer. Cutting down on sun exposure at any age is therefore likely to reduce significantly the number of future solar keratoses or skin cancers that may develop.

The relationship between sunlight exposure and skin cancer is most clear-cut for solar keratoses and squamous cell cancers, almost all of which develop on skin that is constantly exposed, such as the face and backs of the hands. For malignant melanoma, however, such a relationship, although still convincing, is less easy to understand. This type of cancer is more common in fair-skinned people with a large number of moles, particularly unusual ones, and in those who have sunbathed intermittently and burned a lot. In addition, melanomas mostly appear on parts of the body that have been only intermittently in the sun, such as the trunk and lower leg. This suggests repeated bursts of intense sun exposure causing actual sunburn on a number of occasions are likely to be particularly important in melanoma causation.

In addition, we don't fully understand the exact association between sun exposure and basal cell cancers, and other factors besides sunlight again appear to be involved (we don't know why these cancers appear more commonly on some parts of the skin than others); however, the relationship with sun exposure is thought by some to be similar to that for melanoma.

The very strong overall association between sun exposure and skin cancer development suggests that up to 90 per cent of such cancers could be prevented if people took proper steps to protect their skins carefully from sunlight from an early age (see pages 45–6).

WHO IS AT RISK?

People with skin types I, II and III (see page 26), namely all those with fair skins, are most most likely to develop skin photoageing and cancer: the fairer the skin, the greater the risk. Further, people who sunbathe, work outdoors for large parts of their life, enjoy outdoor hobbies, such as cycling, gardening, tennis, cricket or golf, or live in sunny climates at low latitudes, are particularly likely to be affected.

As stated earlier, some people with skin cancer may claim never to have sunbathed or worked outside, and therefore wonder how they developed the condition. In most cases, the answer is that they are very fair-skinned and have been exposed a lot as a child or repeatedly for short periods over many years, usually through routine activities such as walking to and from the office, sitting outside for a sandwich at lunchtime in the summer or gardening. Although not proved conclusively, cigarette smoking may also increase skin cancer risk.

People at risk of melanoma

usually also have a fair skin, although other factors are likely to be important as far as they are concerned. Those with large numbers of moles, particularly oddly shaped ones, and those with a family history of melanoma, are especially liable to develop the condition, particularly if they have sunbathed and burned a lot. Similarly, basal cell cancers appear to be associated with other, as yet unknown, causative factors besides sunlight, and occasionally with a family history of the condition, although fair skin and frequent sun exposure are again likely to be most important. If you wish to know more about any of this, you should arrange to see your family doctor or a dermatologist.

CAN SKIN CANCER BE PREVENTED?

Skin cancers can largely be prevented. It is estimated that over 90 per cent of such lesions are avoidable by reducing your exposure to UV radiation. You can best achieve this by doing the following with this order of priority:

- Tend to undertake outdoor activities, in summer, tropical climates or at altitude, outside the hours of 11:00 to 15:00, namely when the sun is lower in the sky, even on cloudy or cool days. This is even more important if there is a lot of sky visible, or if there are white surfaces, snow or areas of rippling water nearby. If you must sunbathe, do it outside these situations, as the UV intensity is weaker then, even if the weather is hot and sunny, and wear a highly protective sunscreen.

- Wear suitably protective clothing where possible, especially a broad-brimmed hat, a longish-sleeved, loosely fitting, close-weave top, and similar apparel for the legs; in the UK and some other countries, special UV-protective clothing is available, and this may be used instead for greater reliability where desired.

- Routinely use a highly protective sunscreen on exposed skin when outside, particularly between the hours of 11:00 and 15:00 in summer, in the tropics and at altitude. Re-apply such preparations every hour or so, particularly after swimming or exercise.

- This advice is even more important for young children, who have more sensitive skins, are unaware of the implications of excessive sunlight exposure and also have lots of free time available to be outside.

✓ UV radiation-induced skin damage, particularly to cellular DNA, may lead to later skin photoageing and cancer

✓ Virtually everyone regularly exposed to such radiation over many years will develop skin photoageing – a dry, itchy, blotchy, yellowish wrinkling of exposed sites

✓ Some, particularly fair-skinned, people will also develop skin cancer: melanoma occurs not uncommonly in those who are fair and have been badly burned on occasion, and non-melanoma in those exposed consistently over many years

✓ Minimisation of UV radiation exposure will reduce or avoid these conditions

Prevention of sun-induced disorders

As we have seen, you need to be particularly careful when the UV radiation in sunlight is at its most intense. The sensible approach is to adopt a Mediterranean or Mexican lifestyle, tending to stay inside around the middle of the day, and seeking the shade if outside at such times, as well as covering up with suitable clothing and using a highly protective sunscreen; you may, however, enjoy the outdoors relatively harmlessly at other times.

If you're reluctant to take such precautions because you think they stop you from enjoying the sun, you need to realise that, if you don't, you will almost certainly develop the signs of photoageing – a dry, itchy, blotchy, coarse and wrinkled skin. What's more, you are also putting yourself at increased risk of a potentially lethal skin cancer; and both this and photoageing are more likely if you are fair-skinned. All white skins, in fact, although not black or, to a lesser extent, brown ones, are poorly designed to cope with strong UV exposure, and it is most sensible to enjoy being outdoors when the sun is lowish in the sky. Even if the weather is bright and hot, the damaging UVB will be less intense at these times; although UVA will still be around, this is many times less efficient at causing skin damage.

So, during the middle of a summer day, stay inside or else cover up with suitable clothing and routinely use a sun-screen, even if there is a cool breeze or a cloudy sky, and be more relaxed in your precautions for the rest of the time.

Don't forget either that most people in the UK who have indoor jobs get almost half their total sun exposure each year during a single two-week holiday abroad, so you definitely need to be sensible then. However, this does not mean that you cannot enjoy your sunshine holiday as much as before – you just need to take a little extra care!

DRESS, FASHION AND SUN PROTECTION

Until the 1950s, it was relatively common to see people wearing hats – and relatively uncommon to see them sunbathing on the beach. However, changes in fashion and behaviour over the last few decades have meant that we are increasingly exposing ourselves to the summer sun and consequently at greatly increased risk of its harmful effects.

If you are out around midday in the summer, particularly if you have a thinning head of hair, consider wearing a hat, preferably with a broad brim; this will protect both your scalp and your face from much of the sun's harmful radiation. Also try to wear close-weave, loose-fitting cotton or similar clothing to protect your shoulders, back and arms, and something of similar quality to protect your legs. If you are swimming, wind-surfing or sailing, aim to wear at least a T-shirt,

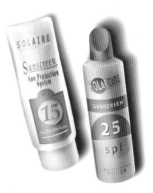

which will provide some sun protection. Unfortunately, however, such shirts are rather less effective when wet than when dry. Perhaps a better choice in such situations is therefore to wear clothing made from specially designed beach-wear fabrics with a high clothing protection factor number stamped on them. These are now available in many department stores for children and young adults, and provide the same UV protection whether wet or dry.

SUNSCREENS AND SUN PROTECTION

Sunscreens are skin creams, lotions, mousses or sprays designed to diminish the risk of sunburn by reducing the amount of UV radiation reaching your skin; they also appear significantly to reduce the risk of skin photoageing and cancer if used properly. Sunblock is also a term used in this regard, but just refers to more powerful sunscreens – sunblocks are

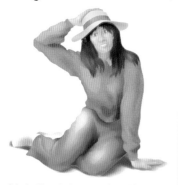

A hat will protect your scalp and face from a great deal of UV radiation.

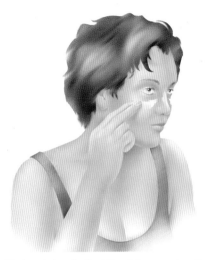

Sunblock works by reflecting UV radiation away from the skin.

generally white creams containing zinc and titanium oxides that act like a sheet of baking foil and reflect the sunlight; in spite of the name, however, they still let some UV radiation through!

However, all these products are effective only if you always apply them carefully before sun exposure, re-apply them every hour or so, and don't think that using them means you can then stay in the sun indefinitely.

There are essentially three types of product: those containing organic chemical substances that absorb UV radiation, those containing fine inert powders that largely reflect it, and combinations of the two. In the UK, most are combinations and provide protection against both UVB and UVA, although relatively less against UVA. However, in other countries this dual effect may not always be present, so check carefully on the packaging. It is now generally agreed that double protection is preferable, although UVB efficacy is certainly more important.

The SPF (sun protection factor) number on the packaging of sunscreens indicates the level of protection against sunburn from UVB and UVA combined, compared with that of unprotected skin; the higher the number, the better the protection, the value in fact indicating approximately the number of times that your skin damage is reduced while wearing the preparation. The degree of UVA protection alone is sometimes defined but less important. It may be designated by a star-rating (* to

****) – again, the more stars the better the protection provided. However, exact UVA protection is not easy to measure and the star ratings are therefore only a guide.

Unfortunately, in many cases, the more effective a sunscreen, the more visible it is on your skin, because the stronger preparations contain reflectant products that are not well absorbed. This means that combining a high SPF with good UVA protection and satisfactory cosmetic qualities may be more expensive, so that the choice you make must depend on what you want from your product (see below); newer formulations are, however, becoming more reasonably priced. In any case, a sunscreen of SPF 15–25 with a good star-rating is usually strong enough for normal use and generally also cosmetically acceptable.

If you are concerned about avoiding sunburn, photoageing and cancer, you need highish levels of protection, say around SPF 15–25 with a high UVA star-rating. In addition, a variety of all-year-round moisturising sunscreen products is now available on the market; these appear worthwhile because the skin changes leading to photoageing and cancer accumulate with levels of UV radiation exposure that are

CHOOSING A SUNSCREEN

When you choose a sunscreen, first select one with good sun protection qualities (see column on the left), then decide which you prefer with respect to your other requirements (see column on the right).

Sun protection
✓ High SPF (15–25)
  (= high sunburning protection)
✓ High star-rating (****)
  or other designation of UVA protection
  (= high UVA protection)

Other considerations
✓ Water-resistance
✓ Blending with your natural skin colour
✓ Ease of application
✓ Acceptable smell
✓ Presence or absence of fragrances or lanolin (some people are allergic to these substances)
✓ Affordability
✓ Acceptable feel
✓ Acceptable appearance

REDUCING YOUR RISK OF SUN-INDUCED SKIN DAMAGE

- Avoid excessive exposure outdoors around midday in summer
- Cover as much of your skin as convenient with suitable clothing when so exposed
- Wear a cosmetically suitable, combined UVB and UVA sunscreen with a high SPF (15–25) and high UVA protection (often designated as a star-rating – * to ****)
- Re-apply the sunscreen every hour or so if you are outdoors for prolonged periods and after swimming, perspiration or exercise
- Consider also using a sunscreen routinely, perhaps incorporated into a moisturiser, on the face and hands, particularly in summer

often insufficient to cause sunburn. In other words, you don't have to burn to accumulate the steady skin damage necessary for significant long-term effects.

Other effective, protective options range from tinted products, which blend in with your skin colour, to brightly coloured preparations designed to look interesting, to water-resistant and hypoallergenic preparations for those with sensitive skins. Ask your pharmacist's advice about the best type for you.

Sunscreens do have occasional side effects, but these are generally not serious; they include quite frequent mild irritation soon after application, particularly around the eyes, and rare allergic itchy rashes; if this happens, change the sunscreen. Most itchy rashes occurring during sunscreen use are not, however, caused by the product, but represent a form of sun-induced rash (see page 58).

Finally, some people use sunscreens to increase the time that they can stay outdoors uncovered without burning, perhaps to achieve a tan, perhaps just for the fun of it. However, although you may well avoid getting burned in this way, you have to accept that such sunscreen use may not necessarily provide enough protection to prevent future skin photoageing, or even skin cancer, especially if you are very fair.

PROTECTION FOR CHILDREN

Children are especially vulnerable to the damaging effects of sunlight for several reasons. First, their skin has had little time to build up gentle tanning and thickening to give a degree of protection and is thus more likely to be damaged. In addition, children don't understand why they should protect their skin by avoiding midday summer sun, wearing hats, covering up, applying sunscreens and so on, so you need to be vigilant on their behalf. What's

WHAT YOU CAN DO TO PROTECT CHILDREN

- Don't expose your baby's skin to direct sunlight and remember that he or she can sometimes burn even if shaded on sunny days.
- Protect even dark-skinned babies, as they too can occasionally burn when young; all young skin needs protection.
- Encourage young children to wear a sunscreen during the summer months, and to apply it carefully themselves. Choose one of the many brands packaged specifically for them with the aim of making it fun. Put this into your child's school bag and enlist the teacher's support where possible to encourage its use before school breaks outdoors.
- Always select products giving high protection (SPF of 15 to 25 with high UVA protection or star-rating) for your child.
- Encourage your child to wear a hat, ideally with some neck protection, during school breaks and when outside in summer.
- Look at the range of specially designed sun-protective clothes for children; these generally carry a high SPF rating, protect much of the body from direct sunlight, and provide the same protection whether wet or dry.
- Set a good example – behave sensibly in the sun yourself and explain to your child why this is necessary.

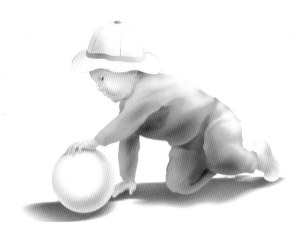

Children are especially vulnerable to the damaging effects of sunlight.

more, they tend to be outside more often than many adults, because they have more time and enjoy the outdoors, for example, during school lunch breaks.

It is estimated that we receive around 50 per cent of our total lifetime sun exposure by the age of 18 – and it is overall lifetime exposure that leads to skin photo-ageing and possible cancer. It follows therefore that the effort involved in minimising your child's exposure while young is very worthwhile, particularly as careful habits developed early are much more likely to remain than those taught later.

By setting an example, and making sure your children understand the dangers of sun exposure, you can lay the foundations for sensible behaviour in the future and help to ensure that they have healthy skins throughout their lives.

KEY POINTS

✓ Taking precautions doesn't mean you cannot enjoy sunshine – you just need to take a little extra care!

✓ Hats and loose fitting clothing afford good protection

✓ Sunscreens and sunblocks reduce the amount of UV radiation reaching your skin

✓ The SPF (sun protection factor) of a sunscreen indicates the level of protection that it offers; the higher the number the greater the protection

✓ Children's skins are relatively sensitive to UV radiation and are more likely to be exposed because of their outdoor habits and lack of scientific understanding

✓ Protect children's skin carefully and teach them good habits for the future

Treatment of sun-induced disorders

No sun-induced skin disorders are particularly easy to treat and it is far better to prevent their development in the first place if possible.

SUNBURN

There is little that can be done to treat the immediate symptoms of this effectively, and nothing at all to stop any associated long-term damage afterwards; however, if you do overdo things somewhat, the following may help a little until natural healing takes place:

- Drink plenty of non-alcoholic fluids and apply a soothing preparation, such as calamine lotion or aqueous cream, to the affected areas; you can buy both over the counter at pharmacies.

- Take aspirin, paracetamol or non-steroidal anti-inflammatory tablets such as ibuprofen in normal doses as soon as possible after exposure, to help ease soreness until the skin has healed. Ibuprofen gel or similar, although not made specifically for sunburn, and local anaesthetic preparations may also help a little. Ask the advice of your pharmacist.

- Stay out of the sun for a few days, until the redness and soreness have fully subsided.

- If your sunburn is severe or widespread – for example, if your skin has blistered significantly or you have symptoms such as shivering, headaches or nausea – you should probably consult a doctor, or in particularly serious cases go to a hospital accident and emergency department. The complications of very severe widespread sunburn can include skin infection and scarring, as well as generalised dehydration, collapse and rarely even death. Over-exposure to the sun can be dangerous!

PHOTOAGEING

If your skin is already affected by photoageing, you may be able to improve its appearance to some extent by using simple moisturising creams regularly to help relieve the associated dryness and smooth out any wrinkles, but you must use them always. In addition, there is some evidence that the daily use of creams containing vitamin A derivatives (so-called retinoids), and in particular Retinova cream containing tretinoin, available on prescription, may slowly reduce irregular pigmentation and smooth out fine wrinkles to a minor extent.

Cosmetic or plastic surgery by an appropriate surgeon can also help in a more invasive, expensive and perhaps risky fashion, in many cases satisfactorily smoothing out wrinkled, sagging areas of skin. Relatively mild, often effective treatments for brown blotchiness and thread veins include cryo-therapy and cold point cautery, generally available from a derma-tologist. If these are not helpful, however, other more aggressive treatments for the same problem are chemical peels and laser therapy, the latter being particularly effective for wrinkles. However, this treatment leaves treated areas extremely red and raw initially for days to weeks, and you will need to take into account the cost and the slight risk of permanent scarring before deciding to go ahead. Discuss it carefully with a derma-tologist or surgeon first.

SKIN CANCER

The treatment of skin cancer depends on its precise type and location on the body. Regardless of which treatment you are offered, you will always be strongly advised to cut down considerably on future sun exposure. The fact that you have had a skin cancer already means that the sun-exposed skin on other parts of your body is also likely to have been significantly damaged over the years, and you are therefore at risk of developing another cancer if you continue exposure to too much sunlight.

Solar (or actinic) keratoses

There is a minor degree of debate among doctors as to whether the treatment of solar keratoses offers enough benefit in terms of reducing future skin cancer risk to be worth doing, as so many older people have them and so few progress to cancer. However, it does appear that at least one to two per cent do advance, especially if the person concerned does not reduce his or her sun exposure from then on, and most people also find them unsightly and itchy or sore. Therefore, it is generally agreed that such lesions should be treated once established and you should consult your doctor if you have any suspicious patches. Treatment usually means the use of cryotherapy (see pages 56–7), which is generally very effective. Cancer cell-killing creams available on prescription may also be recommended on occasion. These must be applied regularly over several weeks, during which they kill off the abnormal but not the normal skin, although they may also make the area unpleasantly red and sore for a few weeks. Staying out of the sun thereafter appears to help prevent the development of new lesions.

Finally, it is most important to have solar keratoses treated if you are on drugs that tend to suppress your immune system, such as cyclosporin or azathioprine (mostly prescribed after organ transplantations but occasionally for other reasons), because these drugs greatly increase the risk that keratoses will progress to skin cancer.

Basal cell cancers

Small basal cell cancers can be treated with cryotherapy (see pages 56–7), but cutting them out surgically or their ablation by radiotherapy is much more reliable for larger ones (see pages 55–6). Sometimes, this type of cancer may come back after treatment, and a similar, but perhaps slightly more aggressive, approach will then be needed to provide a final certain cure. Basal cell cancers do not spread to other parts of the body, except in extraordinarily rare instances, and the only real trouble with them is the way they look and their tendency to erode very slowly into nearby tissues.

Squamous cell cancers

Squamous cell cancers are most often treated by surgery, except sometimes in difficult-to-reach skin sites or in people who are frail, when radiotherapy may be used instead (see pages 55–6); it is relatively unusual for the condition to come back. However, up to about five per cent do reappear or, much more rarely, spread to other parts of the body, such as nearby lymph glands in the neck or armpit, for example, or very occasionally to the lungs, bones or brain. If this should happen, however, further surgery or chemotherapy often discourages further growth. It is generally cancers that have been left for a long time and become particularly large locally that cause problems, although lesions of the lip or ear, or in individuals whose immune system is suppressed by certain illnesses or medications (see pages 62–5), are also relatively likely to spread if not dealt with early. If you have a growth on your skin that you think might be this type of cancer, you should see your doctor soon, so the problem can be dealt with before any chance of spread.

Melanoma

Melanomas are virtually always treated by surgery. They are generally cut out under local anaesthetic and fully and permanently cured. The usual procedure is that any suspicious mole is removed first with a narrow margin of normal skin for careful examination under the microscope. If a melanoma is confirmed, however, a larger area is often removed at a separate visit to ensure that no tumour remains. Occasionally, this may require skin grafting but more often you will just be left with a line scar.

If you have a melanoma, you should discuss the matter in some detail with your dermatologist or surgeon. The vast majority of such tumours are, however, very thin and non-invasive, do not recur and give no further trouble. Nevertheless,

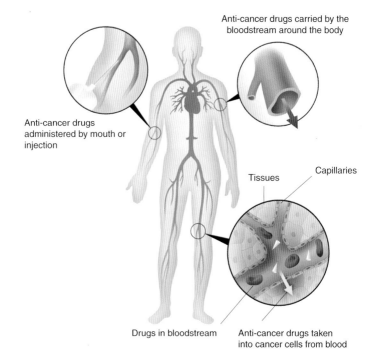

Anti-cancer drugs carried by the bloodstream around the body

Anti-cancer drugs administered by mouth or injection

Tissues

Capillaries

Drugs in bloodstream

Anti-cancer drugs taken into cancer cells from blood

Chemotherapy is particularly useful when cancers have spread from the original tumour to other areas. With this technique, anti-cancer drugs are carried throughout the body by the bloodstream.

some deeper ones do have a risk of recurrence or spread to other areas of the body through the lymph vessels or bloodstream. It is therefore often a good idea to make a further appointment to see your doctor some weeks after your surgery, when you have had time to think, during which period you can make a list of any questions that you want to ask. For example, you might want to be told about your own specific risk of recurrence or spread, or whether the event might alter any future decision to have children, or whether you might conceivably develop another tumour. If necessary, see also 'Useful addresses' for contact details of the Macmillan Nurses, who specialise in the care of people with more persistent melanomas.

After treatment, anyone who has had a melanoma will normally have regular check-ups in the clinic from their dermatologist or surgeon about every six months for five years, or sometimes longer. At these visits, the scar and local lymph nodes will usually be examined for any sign of possible recurrence; usually there isn't any. A cancer that does reappear in the same place is often treated with further surgery, which is frequently successful. If, on the other hand, the condition has spread to the local lymph glands, these can usually also be removed effectively at surgery,

although chemotherapy may be given at this stage to help prevent further dissemination. This is because the drugs used with this technique are able to destroy cancer cells wherever they may be in the body.

Although rare, melanoma is potentially the most aggressively lethal skin cancer; however, early diagnosis and prompt removal are almost always fully curative.

PROCEDURES USED FOR DIAGNOSING AND TREATING SKIN CANCERS

Surgery – the skin biopsy for diagnosis and treatment

You will probably need to undergo a special procedure called a skin biopsy to establish the precise diagnosis of your condition. This is a simple technique that removes part or all of a tumour for microscopic examination to determine what cancer it is and, particularly if large, what treatment is best to dispose of it. Usually, however, the abnormality is fully removed during the biopsy, and the tissue is then just examined to check the diagnosis and that all of the cancer has indeed been taken away. If the margins of the lesion are very close to or impinge on the removed skin edges, however, your doctor may need to excise more tissue to get rid of the cancer cells completely. If the cancer is large, on the other

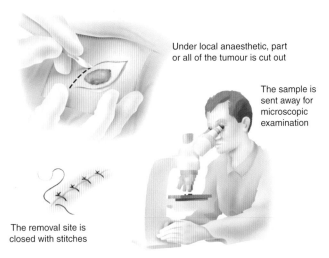

Under local anaesthetic, part or all of the tumour is cut out

The sample is sent away for microscopic examination

The removal site is closed with stitches

A skin biopsy usually establishes the diagnosis of your condition.

hand, or awkward to remove completely because of where it is, only a small piece of skin may be taken at first just for microscopic examination; a further procedure will then probably be planned for later.

The skin biopsy procedure itself is relatively simple and normally requires no special preparation on your part; you can eat and drink normally beforehand, and also as soon afterwards as you wish. Furthermore, it usually takes only between 10 and 30 minutes or so to perform and the local anaesthetic used generally does not cause nausea, drowsiness or other unpleasant effects. As long as you feel comfortable, therefore, there is no real reason not to drive home or go back to work afterwards if you

wish. However, many people prefer to take the day off just in case they find the whole event a strain or in case any minor soreness afterwards is annoying; they may therefore also arrange for someone to drive them home.

You should inform your doctor beforehand if you are on any medication, particularly steroids, aspirin, non-steroidal anti-inflammatory drugs or warfarin, all of which may conceivably interfere with healing or cause increased bleeding during the procedure. You should also alert your doctor if you have ever had an adverse reaction to an anaesthetic, although this is rare, or if you are allergic to any other relevant substances, such as sticking plaster. Finally, you should mention if you have had any heart valve abnormalities or replacements, because you may then require antibiotics at the time of the biopsy.

The local anaesthetic used for the procedure is a generally a liquid gently injected through a fine needle into and around the area to be removed. You can usually briefly feel the sharpness of the needle, some skin areas being more sensitive than others, and often also a little stinging as the anaesthetic goes in, but this rapidly passes and thereafter there should be no discomfort. As the effect then wears off over an hour or so, you may again experience a little soreness, aching or tenderness at the biopsy site, but this is usually mild and can be eased if necessary by taking mild pain relief medication.

After the event, the removal site will usually be closed with stitches and covered with a dressing. All you then have to remember is to keep the affected skin carefully clean and dry. You will probably also have to go back to your doctor four to fourteen, or occasionally more, days later to have the stitches removed. However, if the wound oozes or bleeds more than just slightly after the operation, you may need to see your doctor again sooner, and may perhaps need a pressure pad or further stitch for the wound. If you develop pain or swelling at the site over the next few days, you should again consult your doctor sooner because the area may have become infected, which interferes with healing. If this does happen, a course of antibiotics will usually solve the problem, or else occasionally the stitches may need to be removed early.

Radiotherapy

Although most forms of skin cancer can be cured by surgical removal, occasionally this may not be the best approach, particularly if the lesion is large or in a place that makes removal awkward, or if the person concerned is very old or frail. In these circumstances, therefore, radiotherapy may be used instead; this generally involves the use of superficial X-rays over a short course of treatment to destroy the abnormal cells; in addition, some normal tissue may be damaged and whiteness, superficial scarring or spider veins may therefore occur and persist at the

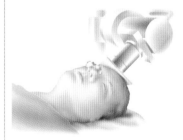

Radiotherapy uses X-rays to destroy cancer cells.

treated site, although generally there are no other important side effects.

Photodynamic therapy

In rare instances, so-called photo-dynamic therapy may be used to treat your skin cancer; this is still an experimental procedure, however, and your doctor will explain it fully to you beforehand if it is being considered. The technique involves the use of a photosensitising chemical called a porphyrin pre-cursor, which is either injected into or applied to the skin, after which it is taken up just by the cancer cells because they are most active. When visible light is then applied to the affected area over a course of treat-ment, it is absorbed by the chemical and destroys the cancer, generally causing a little soreness or burning, but no other problems. However, some people who have this treatment may be advised to avoid daylight for several hours afterwards, as the skin may remain very sensitive to sunburning for that time after the injected drug.

Cryotherapy

For most solar keratoses and some small or superficial basal cell cancers, the preferred treatment is often cryotherapy, sometimes after biopsy to confirm the diagnosis. The technique is relatively simple and involves freezing of the lesion on one or several occasions a few

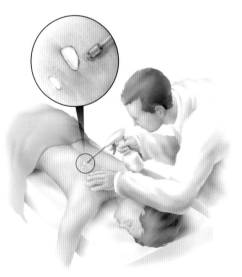

Cryotherapy freezes lesions with a localised spray of liquid nitrogen, generally killing all the cancer cells.

weeks apart with a localised spray of liquid nitrogen. A severe cold injury of around –40°C is inflicted on the cancer or pre-cancer cells which kills them. While the treatment is being given, you will experience a moderate to marked burning feeling, which persists for seconds to minutes, after which the skin will be red for another few minutes to hours, then often blistering or sometimes breaking down over a day or so to form a scab. Thereafter, usually over about a further two weeks, healthy skin forms at the damaged site; it is usually reddish to begin with, but later totally normal. Occasionally, the area may become brownish for some weeks or else very rarely permanently pale, especially if a larger lesion was treated aggressively.

Cryotherapy is generally convenient and effective, being quick, involving relatively modest discomfort and virtually never leaving scars, but still killing any cancer or pre-cancer cells effectively. It does not, however, penetrate very deeply and, any lesion that is large, of uncertain diagnosis or suspected of being aggressive must be excised or treated with radiotherapy to ensure success.

KEY POINTS

✓ Short- and long-term UV-induced damage responds relatively poorly to treatment; prevention is the best approach

✓ Sunburn improves a little with sun avoidance, calamine lotion or cream, and mild pain relief medication

✓ Skin photoageing improves mildly with moisturisers or retinoic acid-containing creams; surgical or laser treatments are now more effective, but expensive and more risky

✓ Skin cancers are virtually always cured by minor surgery or radiotherapy; cryotherapy may be used in mild cases

✓ Delay in diagnosis of skin cancers may lead to cancer spread and the need for major surgery or chemotherapy

Sun-induced rashes

There are some 20 to 30 of these conditions, many of them rare; they are subdivided into groups as described below. Polymorphic light eruption (colloquially called prickly heat) is the most common and is given most attention.

ALLERGIC SKIN REACTIONS TO SUNLIGHT

Polymorphic light eruption

About 10 to 15 per cent of people in the UK have this condition, often incorrectly known as prickly heat because it is caused not by warmth but by UV radiation; about five per cent of Australians, 10 per cent of North Americans and 20 per cent of Scandinavians also have it. More women than men are affected, often from adolescence or early adulthood, although children also develop it occasionally and a few adults in later life as well. Skin type makes little difference, and black and brown skins are quite frequently affected; there may also be a family history of the condition.

Within minutes to hours of exposing your skin to spring or summer sun, an intensely itchy, red, spotty rash, often like goose-flesh, blisters or hives, develops, often only on some exposed areas but usually symmetrically; it frequently doesn't affect the face or backs of the hands. The outbreak generally lasts for a few days to weeks before gradually subsiding, provided that the skin is protected from sunlight. Most people just have the problem on very sunny days, or once or twice at the start of the sunny season, or on holidays abroad, but more severely affected individuals may suffer throughout the whole spring and summer.

The exact cause of polymorphic light eruption is not fully understood, but it seems likely that a

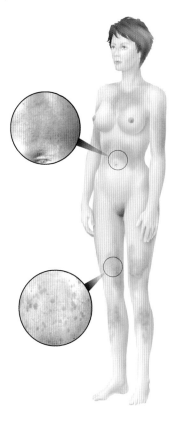

Polymorphic light eruption.

light eruption never consult their doctor; either they have learnt to live with it or they avoid strong sunlight. For others, however, it can be an extremely distressing condition. Nevertheless, it is generally readily treatable and, if you are bothered by it, one or several of the following measures virtually always work:

- Avoid exposing your skin to the sun as much as you can.

- Cover up with suitable clothes whenever possible.

- Use a high SPF sunscreen that gives good UVA protection as well (frequently denoted as a four-star rating), the UVA wavelengths often being particularly important in causing the condition.

- If these measures are not enough, see your GP or, if he or she can't help, ask to see a dermatologist.

genetic predisposition leads some individuals to develop a hyper-sensitivity or allergic reaction to a substance in the skin which is chemically altered by UV radiation and thereby appears foreign to the body. In people who do not have the inherited predisposition, the body apparently fails to react to these altered substances.

Many people with polymorphic

At this stage, the diagnosis must be confirmed because other sunlight-induced conditions (such as lupus, see page 64) may produce similar abnormalities; none is, however, quite like polymorphic light eruption. After this, you may be offered preventive UV photo-therapy, which, in 60 to 90 per cent of cases, stops the rash appearing for several months to a year or two before further treatment may be needed. This therapy comprises a several-week course of twice-weekly, low-dose, artificial UV lamp exposures at the beginning of spring or before a holiday; it is available in many hospitals (see pages 66–8). Paradoxically, such an approach seems to correct the allergic response but is too low in dose to do any harm apart from occasionally inducing the rash temporarily, after which it may still be effective anyway. The treatment is then repeated if necessary, annually, for at least the next few years, after which permanent tolerance may occasionally set in.

If the therapy is unavailable, inconvenient, ineffective or

RARER ALLERGIC REACTIONS TO SUNLIGHT

Chronic actinic dermatitis: a very infrequent condition usually affecting older men, especially those who have had a lot of previous sun exposure, possibly from outdoor hobbies such as gardening. It mostly affects the face, neck and backs of the hands with a persistent eczema, caused and maintained very readily by UV radiation.

Actinic prurigo: a rare, persistent, scratched, spotty, sun-induced rash of the arms, legs and face of children, worse in summer.

Hydroa vacciniforme: a very rare, blistering, scarring, sun-induced eruption of the skin of children, which otherwise behaves in a similar fashion to polymorphic light eruption.

Solar urticaria: a rare, recurrent, nettle rash-like eruption, usually with the hives running together, which comes on within minutes of sunlight exposure, and subsides within an hour or two of covering up.

Treatment for all these conditions includes avoiding sunlight, covering up with appropriate clothing and using a sunscreen, as well as preventive phototherapy, as described above for polymorphic light eruption. If the phototherapy is insufficient, then various specific oral medications may be offered.

unnecessary because of the rarity of your attacks, however, a final, usually very useful treatment is to have a corticosteroid injection or course of tablets, available from your GP or dermatologist, for a few days, as early as possible in an attack, which will usually settle it rapidly. Such treatment may be used up to about every three to four months if required; more frequent or lengthy courses have the potential to cause a gradual build-up of side effects. Brief treatment every now and then rarely causes trouble, indigestion and minimal depression being all that might happen; in this case the medication should be stopped and the effects rapidly disappear. For frequent rashes, UV phototherapy is needed instead.

RARE DNA REPAIR DISORDERS

Xeroderma pigmentosum

Another, extraordinarily rare group of conditions causing sensitivity to the sun is the DNA repair-defective disorders; the most common is xeroderma pigmentosum. This usually causes a strong tendency to sunburn, often with severe blistering after very little sun exposure, and to very early skin photoageing and cancer. This is because people with the condition cannot effectively repair the skin DNA damage caused by UV radiation exposure as a result of inherited defective DNA-repair genes. If you suspect that one of your children may have this, see your doctor; treatment is difficult but not necessarily impossible.

CHEMICALS, DRUGS AND EXCESSIVE SUNLIGHT SENSITIVITY

Porphyria

A group of rare conditions that are frequently aggravated, but not directly caused, by sunlight is the porphyrias. These are predominantly, but not solely, inherited disorders, the most common being porphyria cutanea tarda. This generally affects people of middle age with symptoms of skin fragility, along with scattered, occasional blistering of the sun-exposed skin, usually of the backs of the hands. Such changes occur because porphyrins, the chemical building blocks of the red haemoglobin pigment in blood, accumulate and absorb too much light in the skin, thereby being stimulated into damaging the surrounding tissue. It is therefore important to consult your doctor if this seems to be happening to you because the condition is usually treatable; if nothing is done, however, liver damage may develop in some instances. Just occasionally, excessive sunbed use may also cause a similar condition but this does not lead to liver damage.

A rarer type of porphyria, which causes a much greater degree of sun sensitivity, is known as erythropoietic protoporphyria (EPP). This generally starts in early childhood and is associated with a very severe, painful, burning skin sensation after UV radiation and visible violet light exposure within minutes of being outside in the summer. Again this happens because excessive porphyrin in the skin absorbs the radiation, leading to nearby tissue damage. If a child is too young to tell you that his or her skin hurts, the only sign of this condition might be crying whenever the child is in the sun. Any youngster who reacts in this way should be seen by the family doctor and if necessary by a dermatologist, in case EPP may be the cause. Treatment is difficult but not always impossible.

Reactions to drugs and creams

There are a large number of oral medicines and skin preparations that can increase skin sensitivity to UV radiation in a variety of ways. Most often they cause a sunburn-like inflammation, or sometimes blistering, of skin that has been exposed to the sun, but there may be other problems such as a burning sensation without a rash,

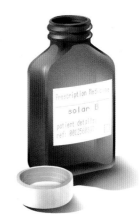

skin fragility with scattered blisters, eczema or, occasionally, nail abnormalities. Generally, the sensitivity develops within days to weeks of starting a new medication, unless perhaps this is in winter and you don't see much sun for some time; spring is then the time that the trouble usually starts.

Common medications causing such sensitivity are listed in the box on page 63, but there are many others, so if you think that your skin is affected as described after starting a new drug you should consult your doctor. However, many people can take most of these medications without developing sun sensitivity, and those who do often experience only a mild reaction.

The treatment of drug photo-sensitivity is by changing the drug, restricting sunlight exposure, using a sunscreen regularly, or in some cases just taking the medication at night if medically appropriate.

DRUGS THAT MAY CAUSE PHOTOSENSITIVITY

Medical condition	Photosensitising drug (generic or scientific name)
High blood pressure (hypertension)	Amiloride Bendrofluazide Chlorothiazide Frusemide Nifedipine
Depression/anxiety	Amitriptyline Doxepin Imipramine Chlorpromazine Haloperidol Dothiepin
Pain	Naproxen Piroxicam
Bacterial infections/acne	Doxycycline Oxytetracycline Minocycline Sulphamethoxazole Isotretinoin
Diabetes	Chlorpropamide Tolbutamide
Heart disease	Amiodarone Captopril Quinidine
Epilepsy	Carbamazepine
Used in cosmetics	Fragrances, particularly bergamot oil, sandalwood, lavender

Note: pharmaceutical manufacturers give their particular formulations of drugs trade or brand names, in addition to the approved generic or scientific names, which are the ones listed above. If you suffer from any of the conditions in the table and are taking a medication for it, you should look for the generic/scientific name of the substance on the packaging or the leaflet inside (usually in smallish letters!), to check if it is on this list.

SKIN CONDITIONS NOT CAUSED BUT AGGRAVATED BY SUNLIGHT

There are many skin conditions that are not actually caused by sunlight but which may sometimes be aggravated by it, although some are more likely to improve in most individuals after exposure. Some people with eczema, for example, which is mostly improved by sunlight, find that the sun makes their skin itch more or otherwise makes the eczema worse, even in cool conditions. However, it is more common for heat (from the sun or a fire, for example) to have this effect and, if this happens to you, you may need specialist investigations to determine which sunlight component is actually responsible. Other conditions that may also be aggravated by sun exposure include acne and psoriasis, although again many people who have these find that their skin improves in summer.

No one knows exactly why these conditions are made worse by sunlight in some people, but UV radiation may perhaps alter various skin immune processes causing the diseases, or else sometimes add further sunburn-like inflammation to an already angry and sensitive skin.

The main approach to therapy is to have treatment for the underlying condition, as well as cutting down your exposure to sunlight, and being scrupulous about applying a sunscreen. Sometimes courses of low-dose preventive phototherapy, as for polymorphic light eruption, may also be helpful, except in people who have lupus (see below), when the condition may instead be made worse.

Lupus

This is a disorder best known for its hallmark, if rather rare, abnormality of a fixed, butterfly-shaped, redness of the nose and cheeks, supposedly giving patients' faces a wolf-like look (hence the word *lupus*, which is Latin for wolf). Much more common as far as its light sensitivity is concerned, however, are flat, scaly, slightly sore red patches, apparently induced by the UVB radiation in sunlight, on other exposed sites. This may be the sum total of the condition, although rarely internal abnormalities such as sore joints or a generalised feeling of being unwell may also occur, again sometimes worsened by sun exposure. The condition is also known to be associated with various immunological abnormalities, and one theory of how the rash itself is caused is that cutaneous DNA is changed by the UVB in sunlight to a sufficient extent to cause an allergic skin reaction, similar to that postulated for polymorphic light eruption.

Treatment of the disorder and rash consists of sun avoidance, the use of strong sunscreens and the application of steroid creams; in addition, a variety of oral medications may also be necessary in severe cases, such as certain anti-malarial drugs, oral steroids, immunosuppressive drugs or even rarely thalidomide. Sometimes the condition may also gradually settle spontaneously.

Vitiligo and albinism

Vitiligo and albinism are both associated with a lack of the protective pigment, melanin, in the skin. They appear as white patches or a pallor all over the body respectively, with a marked tendency to easy sunburning of the affected areas. The best advice is to minimise exposure to strong sunlight, cover the affected sites as much as possible with appropriate clothing, and use a high factor sunscreen regularly on all the exposed abnormal skin. Naturally fair-skinned people who have vitiligo will find that protecting the skin as much as possible in this way also helps to prevent the normally pigmented sites from tanning, and so keeps the contrast between normal and abnormal areas less noticeable. Albinos, on the other hand, need to be especially vigilant as they can also develop skin cancer relatively easily if careless in the sun, whereas people with vitiligo usually seem not to, for reasons as yet poorly understood. Albinism is present from birth and is unfortunately untreatable; vitiligo, however, sometimes responds, regrettably often only temporarily, to regular applications of steroid creams or lotions to the affected patches, or else phototherapy, both over a number of months.

Melasma

Melasma, or chloasma as it is also known, is a condition that most often affects young and middle-aged women; it is characterised by a patchy brown melanin pigment discoloration, usually of the face, particularly the temples, cheeks and upper lip, but occasionally of other skin. The exact cause is not known, although a genetic tendency and the female hormone oestrogen seem to predispose to the condition. Other factors apparently involved in triggering it are perfumed substances applied to the affected areas and, most particularly, sun exposure. Some girls first develop the problem around puberty, but the condition is most common after a woman starts taking the oral contraceptive pill (which contains oestrogen) or becomes pregnant, which markedly increases oestrogen levels. The discoloration then generally tends to fade once the pill is stopped or the baby is born; it also helps to minimise sun exposure where possible and to use a sunscreen. Skin preparations containing hydroquinone, such as FadeOut, available over the counter at pharmacists, may gradually decrease the colour as well, if used regularly over several months. Skin irritation, allergy and theoretically, after continual use for months or years, an extremely rare orangey discoloration called ochronosis can result from using FadeOut, although this is a relatively weak preparation, and trouble is therefore most unlikely. Like all medications, however, it should be used in strict accordance with the instructions and if you experience problems you should discontinue its use and seek medical advice.

TREATING SKIN CONDITIONS WITH UV RADIATION (PHOTOTHERAPY)

Although UV radiation is generally harmful to the skin in the long term, there are a number of rashes that can be greatly alleviated, albeit usually only temporarily, by its use as a medical treatment. Such conditions may or may not actually be caused by sunlight, but those most likely to respond are psoriasis, eczema, vitiligo and polymorphic light eruption, although a whole host of others may sometimes do so as well. When used in this specific way, the benefits of UV radiation in a particular individual are considered to outweigh the potential risks, even though the treatment does inevitably involve some overall damage to the skin. The situation is discussed in some detail with the patient beforehand and the treatment, which can be used only for a limited period in total because of the potential build-up of side effects, is not used without the patient's consent.

There are two main types of this UV radiation treatment:

- UVB phototherapy, which is given alone, as either so-called broad- or narrow-band UVB, which refers in each case to the breadth of the wavelength spectrum emitted by the lamp.

- Psoralen and UVA photochemotherapy (PUVA), which is a combination of a photosensitising medication called psoralen with broad-band UVA exposure.

UVA radiation without the psoralen, which is broadly what many, particularly older, sunbeds deliver, is usually many times less effective at treating skin diseases than either UVB or PUVA, but still damaging overall to the skin, and you should not therefore generally use self-therapy with these devices as a substitute for the medically supervised approach.

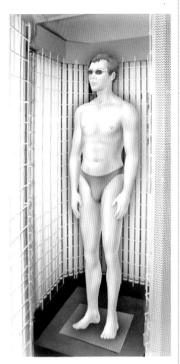

Phototherapy.

Before your doctor decides to offer you phototherapy for any skin condition, he or she will carefully assess you to make sure that to all intents and purposes it will be relatively safe. You will therefore be asked whether you are on any drugs or medications that might increase your UV sensitivity, whether you have had much previous sun exposure and whether you have ever had conditions such as polymorphic light eruption or skin cancer. Your doctor will then explain the advantages and possible risks of the treatment, which include a small chance of burning, and a very gradually increasing risk of photoageing and skin cancer if the therapy should by chance need to be continued over a number of years. These risks are, however, now fairly precisely documented and the radiation doses recorded accurately to ensure safety. The twin aims of medical supervision are clearly to keep each treatment dose below that which might cause sunburn and to ensure that your cumulative (or lifetime) dose is as low as possible overall, so as to minimise the risk of long-term problems.

It is not known for certain how phototherapy improves those conditions that are responsive to it. However, psoriasis and eczema seem to be disorders in which the skin immune system is overactive, thereby causing an inflammation leading to the characteristic rash. Phototherapy appears to modify this response, probably by damaging skin immune cell DNA in the first instance, which thereby impedes various subsequent immunological pathways. In addition, it may also slow down normal, although in psoriasis excessive, epidermal basal cell proliferation; in this way, at least in psoriasis, it may help to reduce the skin overgrowth characteristic of the disease; again, it probably does this by its effect on cellular DNA, this time in the basal cells.

In vitiligo, another disorder that is sometimes responsive to phototherapy, UV radiation exposure again probably damps down abnormal immune activity affecting the skin tanning cells (melanocytes) – very possibly a major causative factor in vitiligo – while also stimulating melanin production in those melanocytes still functioning normally. However, phototherapy is by no means always effective in this condition, many individuals responding too slowly or poorly, whereas others relapse steadily and need continuing treatment; the long-term risks of the therapy may then outweigh the benefits. In practice, therefore, it seems that phototherapy is most suited to vitiligo patients with dark skins and relatively few and small affected patches, particularly on the face or trunk.

Finally, the photosensitivity disorder, polymorphic light eruption, probably an immunologically mediated condition as well, also responds, in this case usually very satisfactorily, to short preventive courses of phototherapy, as already described on page 56.

KEY POINTS

✓ There are a host of sun-induced skin disorders that affect only some people; polymorphic light eruption (prickly heat) and drug photosensitivity are the most common

✓ Polymorphic light eruption (prickly heat) responds very well, if care in the sun and sunscreens are not sufficient, to short courses of low-dose preventive phototherapy or, alternatively, to occasional short courses of steroid tablets or injections

✓ UV phototherapy is used under medical supervision for a number of skin disorders, often very successfully; it does, however, damage the skin slowly, in the same way as sunlight, so it is used only if its benefits are considered to outweigh the risks

Do I really need to worry about sun exposure in the UK?

Yes. Between about April and September in the middle of the day, UV radiation levels in the UK can be almost as high as those in the Mediterranean; the only real differences are that they do not persist for so long and the brightness and warmth of sun, unimportant as far as skin damage is concerned, may be much less, so making the sun seem less dangerous. This means that you can burn almost as easily at around midday on a British beach as you can on a Spanish one. If therefore you spend a fair amount of time outside during the summer months in Britain – playing sport or gardening, for example – or if you have a job that means you are outside for much of the year, you can easily get enough sun to cause skin cancer, particularly if you are fair, and certainly enough to cause photo-ageing, without ever going abroad.

What if I want to get a tan?

You can't sunbathe without causing damage to your skin, however slowly or carefully you build up a tan, so it's better not to aim for this at all. However, if you have a brown or black skin, you are unlikely to do much harm, but you may not then want to tan! It is a personal choice for you to make, but you should certainly be aware of the risks of sunbathing so that you can make an informed decision.

Sunbathing is at its most dangerous for everyone, but most particularly for fair-skinned people, when the sun is high in the sky – whatever the weather; it is thus relatively safe to sit outside either early or late in the day when the sun is low, even if still warm or bright. Therefore, whether at home or abroad, avoid the sun in the middle of the day where possible, wear suitable clothing to cover you when outside, and regularly use a sunscreen of SPF 15 to 25. You should also realise that a suntan is actually a response to skin cell DNA injury caused by UV radiation. However, this again applies much more to fair-skinned people, and the deeper the tan in such people, the greater the skin damage that has been caused, and thus the higher the risk of skin photoageing and cancer in the future.

It is also important to realise that melanoma, although previously relatively rare, has become increasingly common, and that it is a potentially very serious form of cancer that can be fatal. It is now one of the major causes of death in people in the 26- to 35-year-old age group. There is also a lot of evidence to suggest that it is repeated bouts of sunburn, which are most likely to happen when you're sunbathing on holiday, that are particularly important in causing this type of cancer, particularly again in fair-skinned people.

If you want to have a tan, therefore, there is only one way that you can get it safely and conveniently and that is to use a fake tanning preparation! These days, as well as being safe, they can give you a virtually perfect imitation of the real thing.

Nevertheless, if you are going to sunbathe anyway, start with short periods of exposure over a few minutes and gradually build up; also use a sunscreen of moderately high protection factor, say 10–15, and stick with that because, if you do burn, it spoils your tan anyway. Good luck!

Is it safe to use a sunbed?

Sunbeds emit radiation generally very similar to that in midday summer sunlight and therefore have largely the same effects, so you should avoid them. This is because, by using them, you are really just damaging yourself without even being able to enjoy the outdoors at the same time! However, most dermatologists agree that banning them is as inappropriate as banning cigarettes or alcohol; people should rather be made aware of their potential dangers, so they can make an informed choice about using them.

Whether you use the older type of sunbed which emits predominantly UVA radiation, or the more modern ones with UVB and UVA together, the effect in terms of skin damage is very similar to that from tanning in the sun. This means that you are risking the same sort of skin damage, which may sometimes be severe and has even, occasionally, been fatal!

There is also a risk of all the

following problems when you use a sunbed, just as there is when you sunbathe: polymorphic light eruption, lupus, melasma and drug photosensitivity in the short term, and, in the long term, skin ageing and non-melanoma cancer, as well as an unusual form of increased skin fragility. Although the risk of melanoma from sunbed use has not yet been precisely quantified, it seems likely that this is also increased and people with unusual or large numbers of moles should not use a sunbed at all, just as they should not sunbathe. All in all, sunbeds overall are very similar to sunlight in their potential to cause skin damage and should be avoided. If you do use one, however, you may get away with it, but you should use it for no more than 20 sessions a year to keep the risk at least moderate.

Is it a good idea to use a sunbed for just two to three weeks a year before holidays to get a bit of a tan and so avoid burning when I get there?

No, it isn't a good idea to use a sunbed in this way because the damage that you do outweighs the value of any tan or protection that you might achieve, which is virtually always minimal anyway, and equivalent only to a sunscreen of SPF 2–4. Better to use a fake tan and a sunscreen on holiday.

Can sunlight harm my eyes?

Yes, sun exposure is associated with a number of eye problems, including particularly cataracts. For this reason, people having phototherapy for the treatment of skin disease (see pages 66–8) must wear sunglasses; such cataracts occur with long-term exposure over the years. You may also get very sore eyes from severe exposure to bright sunlight, particularly in snow, a condition called snow blindness. Looking directly at the sun for more than a few seconds may cause permanent loss of sight! Ideally you should wear sunglasses on a summer's day to protect your eyes, while of course protecting your skin; however, make sure you buy sunglasses that give you good protection against both UVB and UVA.

If I wear prescription spectacles will this magnify the harmful effect of UV radiation on my eyes?

No. Clear glass or plastic normally absorbs virtually all UV radiation, certainly all the UVB, although obviously allowing visible light to penetrate. You therefore need take no major precautions when wearing prescription spectacles, unless the light is very bright, in which case for comfort you would do best to wear sunglass attachments or else buy prescription sunglasses.

I know I don't get a suntan from sitting in front of the telly or my PC at work, but am I still at risk from UV radiation?

No, there is no risk from either of these because they do not emit this radiation.

I am of Afro-Caribbean origin and have a very dark skin. Do I need to take any precautions against the sun? Should I be careful with my children in sunlight? Am I at the same risk of photoageing as a fair-skinned person?

You need to take only moderate precautions for yourself at the beginning of summer or a sunny holiday, just to stop early burning, although photoageing certainly does still occur over the years in dark skin and you should thus take care if you wish to avoid that; skin cancer essentially does not occur, however. On the other hand, dark-skinned babies can sometimes burn relatively easily and should therefore be carefully protected until older as described in this book.

I seem to have to put a lot of suncream on my skin to cover it properly. Do these chemicals get absorbed into my body and if so can they do me any harm?

No, careful studies suggest that they do not harm you; however, it is probably wise not to use them excessively in babies up to about the age of six months, by which time their skins have generally become fully mature, although there is no definite evidence that such use is damaging.

Useful addresses

British Association of Dermatologists
19 Fitzroy Square
London W1P 5HQ
Tel: 020 7383 0266
Fax: 020 7388 5263
Email: admin@bad.org.uk
Website: www.skinhealth.co.uk

This association represents dermatologists throughout the country. It also provides members of the public with a list of dermatologists in their area, if required, but does not recommend specific doctors. To consult a dermatologist, it is generally necessary to be referred by a general practitioner.

British Association of Plastic Surgeons (BAPS)
Royal College of Surgeons
35–43 Lincoln's Inn Fields
London WC2A 3PN
Tel: 020 7831 5161
Fax: 020 7831 4041
Email: secretariat@baps.co.uk
Website: www.baps.co.uk

Cancer Research Campaign
6–10 Cambridge Terrace
Regents Park
London NW1 4JL
Tel: 020 7224 1333
Fax: 020 7487 4310
Email: cancerinfo@crc.org.uk
Website: www.crc.org.uk

Funds research into cancer and education. Provides information to people with cancer and their carers.

Cancerlink
11–21 Northdown Street
London N1 9BN
Freephone: 0800 808 0000
Freephone (Asian language line): 0800 590415; Freephone (Mac helpline for young people): 0800 591028

Provides information and emotional support for people with cancer and their families. It is a resource to over 500 cancer support and self-help groups throughout Britain. Provides training and advice for people setting up support groups.

Eczema Society
163 Eversholt Street
London NW1 1BU
Information: 020 7388 3444
Admin: 020 7388 4097
Fax: 020 7388 5882
Website: www.eczema.org

Health Development Agency
Trevelyan House
30 Great Peter Street
London SW1P 2HW
Tel: 020 7222 5300

Imperial Cancer Research Fund
PO Box 123
Lincoln's Inn Fields
London WC2A 3PX
Tel: 020 7242 0200
Fax: 020 7269 3100
Website: www.icnet.uk

Provides information on cancer to anyone who wants it.

Macmillan Cancer Relief
Anchor House
15–19 Britten Street
London SW3 3TZ
Information: 0845 601 6161
(9.30am–7.30pm Mon–Fri)
Tel: 020 7351 7811
Fax: 020 7376 8098
Website: www.macmillan.org.uk

A national charity dedicated to improving the quality of life for people with cancer and their families. It funds Macmillan Nursing Services for home care, and hospital and hospice support. Financial help may also be given.

Marie Curie Cancer Care
28 Belgrave Square
London SW1X 8QG
Tel: 020 7235 3325
Fax: 020 7823 2380
Website: www.mariecurie.org.uk

Runs Marie Curie nursing homes and provides a community nursing service day and night. Involved also in research and the education of health professionals in cancer care and prevention.

Psoriasis Association
7 Milton Street
Northampton NN2 7JG
Tel.: 01604 711129
Fax: 01604 792894

Provides information on all aspects of psoriasis, as well as promoting research. It also produces a journal three times a year and organises an annual conference on psoriasis.

Vitiligo Society
125 Kennington Road
London SE11 6SF
Information: 0800 018 2361
Tel: 020 7840 0855
Fax: 020 7 840 0866
Email: all@vitiligosociety.org.uk
Website: www.vitiligosociety.org.uk

Provides information on all aspects of vitiligo, produces a regular journal and organises meetings and events for members with the condition.

Index